Sex and the Breast

Love, Health, and Evolution

VALERIE ROBINSON

BALBOA.
PRESS

A DIVISION OF HAY HOUSE

Balboa Press books may be ordered through booksellers or by contacting:

Balboa Press
A Division of Hay House
1663 Liberty Drive
Bloomington, IN 47403
www.balboapress.com
1 (877) 407-4847

Because of the dynamic nature of the Internet, any web addresses or links contained in this book may have changed since publication and may no longer be valid. The views expressed in this work are solely those of the author and do not necessarily reflect the views of the publisher, and the publisher hereby disclaims any responsibility for them.

The author of this book does not dispense medical advice or prescribe the use of any technique as a form of treatment for physical, emotional, or medical problems without the advice of a physician, either directly or indirectly. The intent of the author is only to offer information of a general nature to help you in your quest for emotional and spiritual well-being. In the event you use any of the information in this book for yourself, which is your constitutional right, the author and the publisher assume no responsibility for your actions.

Any people depicted in stock imagery provided by Getty Images are models, and such images are being used for illustrative purposes only. Certain stock imagery © Getty Images.

Print information available on the last page.

ISBN: 978-1-9822-0814-1 (sc)
ISBN: 978-1-9822-0815-8 (e)

Balboa Press rev. date: 07/17/2018

Dedication

For Stew forever

Acknowledgment

THANKS TO THE MANY people whose writing and research I refer to in my book. I especially appreciate the feedback I received from the scientific journal, *Medical Hypotheses*, which previously published my article on some of the same topics I treat here. I am indebted to Case Western Reserve University for the use of both the Health Sciences Library and the Kelvin Smith Library and to Cleveland State University for the use of its library. Looking back, I am grateful to the many teachers and professors who taught me well throughout my life. And lastly, I thank my husband, Stewart, for his patience and support. His commitment to equality and justice has always inspired me.

Contents

Introduction
A unique feminine way of sex

SEXISM, OR DISCRIMINATION AGAINST women, remains alive at
the most basic level – the neglected study of the female body. While
human society is conversant with vast new computer technologies,
we are content to live with the notion that female sexuality is
"mysterious" or difficult to comprehend. Part of the problem is the
failure to examine the complexity of women's sexuality – essentially
a devaluation of our health – perpetuating a vision of a permanent
male dominated society in which women do not control our own
bodies. The erotic nature of the female breast is rarely researched,
with the result that woman's sexuality is today as misunderstood
and tabooed as ever, and the possible connection of breast sex to
breast health is overlooked. Breast cancer is a killer of women, yet
there is no comprehensive health initiative to investigate women's
sexual use of the breast, an acknowledged practice around the world.
The feminine use of the breast for sex is an ancient practice that
defines a unique feminine way of sex – knowledge of which is passed
from woman to woman outside the realm of academe and medicine.
There is a possible moral dimension to the silence about breast sex.
Recognizing that the famous metaphor of *Genesis*, "forbidden fruit,"
is a veiled reference to woman's breasts, one perceives that breast

sex is condemned by Western religion as the sin of Adam and Eve, no doubt because of woman's instigation and pleasure in it. But if you look with enough persistence, you will find cultural data that indicate that breast sex as a means of attaining female sexual pleasure and orgasm has been practiced in many societies around the world.

Taking its impetus from the work of an exceptional person, Dr. Timothy Murrell, the present book is about female sexuality, specifically sexuality of the breast, its origins and practice and its implications for women's well being and happiness. Dr. Timothy G. C. Murrell, writing in the 1990s, was an Australian physician concerned about the loss of functionality of the human female breast and how this lack of use might be instrumental in the origin of breast cancer. During his tenure at the medical school of Adelaide University, South Australia, he wrote several papers in which he promoted a program of women's self-help that he felt had the potential to reduce the risk of breast cancer.[1,2] His recommendations to women notably included using the breasts sexually in conjunction with a partner. His theory is that nipple stimulation works to relieve the breasts of damaging carcinogens that collect there. He believed that not only the environment, but behavior has a part in causing breast cancer, and he felt that his observations in clinical cases at Adelaide University over the course of 15 years of teaching general medical practice gave credence to his theory. His interest in medical sociology led him to study the function of the breast in several cultures. He also lectured on the positive influence of sex on health and longevity.

We know that the breast provides an undeniable turn-on for the interested man, but, for a woman, what is the sexual meaning, specifically for her, of her breasts? This book is about women's sexuality, and as such it has links to the work of Shere Hite[3] and Naomi Wolf.[4] But whereas Hite's focus is the clitoris, and Wolf's is the vagina, the focus here is the breasts, especially a woman's sexual use of her breasts. The custom of women using their breasts during climactic lovemaking is a cultural phenomenon – not prevalent in every society today, but it may have been universal or near universal in the past. The use of the breast for sexual pleasure is perhaps more characteristic of simpler societies, but it is important to consider that this cultural style of sexuality may be vital to women's health today. This way of sex is sometimes thought of as preliminary only, and male initiated, as in the dating ritual of petting, but there is more to it than the cursory satisfaction of male interest, and it is critical to understand why.

The theory here is that there is a particular woman's way of relating sexually, involving the breasts, which is implicated in the beginnings of modern human culture, that is, *Homo sapiens* culture. It is a way in which women enjoy sex equally with men, and yet have a distinctive experience of their own that is not just a replica of the male experience and certainly different from that of the lower mammalian female. This is cultural sexuality and it implicates the female breast in the beginnings of love and the family. I believe that love between the sexes and the pair-bond first occurred with the appearance of breast sex or "sexual breast love", accompanied by highly climactic sex, starting from the beginning of modern humanity. That is the time when ancestral women acknowledged the erotic potential of the breast and began to use their discovery to establish intimate relationships and innovative communication with men – a new way of sexual and social behavior. The resultant increase in the positive emotions fostered human cooperation, cognition, and the development of the species. These ideas are treated in "Support For the Hypothesis that Sexual Breast Stimulation Is An Ancestral Practice and A Key to Understanding Women's Health" published in *Medical Hypotheses*.[5]

Biologically speaking, the neurotransmitter oxytocin, known as the bonding hormone, is implicated in sexual arousal and orgasm and also in pair bonding. Sexual arousal and orgasm are highly associated with breast sex, as described in various cultural studies that will be looked at further on. The pair-bond is generally thought to be the basis of the human family, the foundational cultural institution of humanity – hence the advent of the cultural practice of breast sex with its attendant bonding hormone, oxytocin, may have been highly significant in the establishment of the family.

Understanding breast sex is made difficult because its practice is not readily admitted – women are reticent on the subject – but also because of the reluctance of doctors and biologists to study the topic. Human sexuality, for those who have a highly credentialed reputation to maintain, has remained a somewhat tabooed field of research. But there are investigators who have undertaken an exploration of the topic, and achieved some acclaim for breaking new ground in the area. With perseverance, adequate documentation can be found to begin to examine the fascinating story of breast sex and cultural sexuality.

Alfred Kinsey, writing in 1953, believed that while sexual breast activity arouses the male, its erotic significance for the female is over-rated.[6] This is an astounding conclusion when one considers that the act of breast play occurs in a large percentage of married couples as ascertained by Kinsey himself, certainly indicating mutual interest, assuming of course that coercion is not the norm in marriage.

Breasts are often thought of as sexual attractants for men, but their basic biological and sexual function for women has not been well researched. The exception is the work of Masters and Johnson on human sexuality, and the scientific literature on oxytocin, sometimes called the love hormone, and its increase in the body with breast stimulation; but even here, more information is needed. The importance of further investigation is that with more knowledge about the female breast, the high incidence of breast cancer can possibly be lowered, and women can appreciate the part the breasts play in our complex sexuality. And of course there is the pleasure that such knowledge can bring.

There are definite indications that breast eroticism may represent an ancestral form of women's sexuality. Apropos of this, in their classic book of 1951, *Patterns of Sexual Behavior*, the authors Ford and Beach named thirteen preliterate societies in which it was reported that woman's breast arousal by a sexual partner accompanies intercourse, and they noted that this is a uniquely human practice.[7] A uniquely human practice must arise at some time in human history or prehistory. When and how did this happen? In the present attempt to look at this phenomenon, breast sex is reviewed in various cultures around the world. Several aspects of the sexual breast are looked at, including the breast in courtship, in marriage, in dress, and more. And the work of Masters and Johnson, and the literature on oxytocin are presented as scientific evidence of the eroticism of the human female breast and its potential for sexual use.

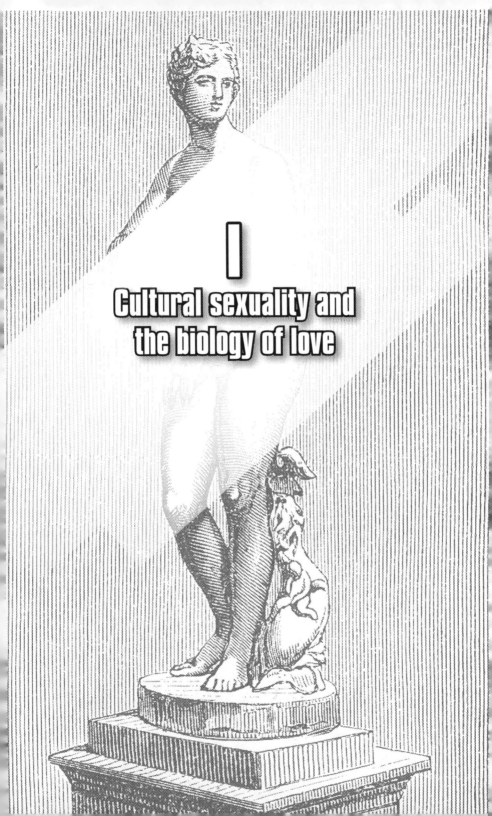

I
Cultural sexuality and the biology of love

1

The sexual breast

IN THE CASE OF the human female, infants are not the only ones to have a happy relationship with her breasts. Her breasts and nipples are mouthed and fingered by mates and lovers as well, providing pleasure to both woman and man and establishing intimacy. What is the basis of this pleasure that a woman feels? When a female mammal's breasts are suckled by her young to obtain nourishment, it is a pleasurable experience for the mother as well as for her offspring. In her book, *A History Of The Breast*, Marilyn Yalom quotes a French doctor of the 16th century, Ambroise Paré (1509-1590), with reference to the joy a woman feels while nursing her child, to which he gives a biological explanation: "There is a sympathetic connection between breasts and the womb; as the breast is tickled, the womb is aroused and feels a pleasurable titillation."[1] According to the doctor, this uterine sensation provides an incentive to the mother to nurse her infant. The deep link between the breasts and the uterus or womb, was appreciated in the 1500s.

The sexual reality of a woman's breasts has been depicted in literature and art, sometimes in graphic ways. Yalom explores the eroticism of the breast in her work mentioned above, which includes literary and artistic references to the sensual breast – a book worth reading for her scholarship on the subject. Recently, two short stories notably describe sexual breast love, the act having serious implications for the main characters. In both *Landfill*, a story written by Joyce Carol Oates in 2006,[2] and *Town of Cats*, a piece by Haruki Murakami from 2011,[3] there are pivotal allusions to breast sex, and the final outcomes of these literary tales are influenced by it. But scientific writing on the erotic breast is another matter. While it is commonly accepted that for a man, a woman's breasts are sexually exciting, with abundant literature attesting to this, there is not much exploration of the fact that attention to her breasts can bring pleasure to a woman, and that she may invite this attention. What is this power of the breast in romantic relationships, and what is its scientific explanation?

To have sex while presenting the breast for sexual enjoyment is a behavior unique to the human female according to the acclaimed authors Ford and Beach in their 1951 book, *Patterns of Sexual Behavior*.[4] No other primate species practices sexual breast love, that is, uses the breast as a means of achieving sexual fulfillment and greater sociality, and it is conjectured here that the uniqueness of the act may implicate it in the origin of our species, *Homo sapiens*. The concept behind this book is that the female offering of the breast to the adult male, and its use for the pleasure of both, was the fundamental cultural act of the first modern humans: cultural sexuality. It was adopted by the group and passed on to succeeding generations. It enabled female orgasm to readily occur during copulation, fostering intimacy and a positive emotional bond, that is, love, between male and female.

This concept is about the erotic power of the female breast and the novel human sexual practices surrounding the breast before and during intercourse. These practices can be documented from around the world. For now, the assessment of anthropologist Paul Gebhard, writing in *Human Sexual Behavior* in 1971, is noteworthy.[5] He says that the male use of the hand on the female breast is universal, but that while the male mouth on the female breast has been recorded for some societies, and is used in the United States by informed people, anthropological data are not complete. There are however, enough anthropological accounts to show that these acts are in fact prompted by women's desire, and are used during intercourse and foreplay around the world in a type of sexual behavior that is not seen among the lower mammals, even in our closest animal relatives, the chimpanzee and bonobo.

Chimpanzees walk away from the sex act as if emotion were absent. For humans, sex can involve conscious desire, love, and other positive emotions which arise with the intense sexual and social pleasure of cultural mating involving the breast. Women, 200,000 years ago or so, upon discovering the erotic and emotional power of breast sex, made it a key to the evolution of humanity. Women's discovery and cultural maintenance of sexual breast love, with the cooperation of men, changed human culture and sociality forever.

Compared to the non-human way of more or less perfunctory genital intercourse, cultural sexuality is a highly intimate and exciting way of relating between the sexes, and is especially pleasing for the female. Woman constituted herself as man's equal when she began to insist on sexual breast love. The inception of this way of better sex meant better reproduction. The human race has prospered in numbers compared to our cousins the chimpanzees and bonobos – perhaps one of the reasons that humans are sometimes called the sexiest animals.

Cultural sexuality can be linked to other changes as well. The mammary way of female orgasm led to a common ground of mutual good feelings and a high level of interdependency in which the sexually cooperating pair learned to work to provide pleasure to each other and to coordinate their actions. Because of the new closeness and reliance on each other, they gained the ability to perceive and appreciate their own and the other's mental states, including the ability to recognize the other's intentions. This is sometimes called "theory of mind." According to a study done in Japan by Yuge, levels of self and other perception are interrelated, and the degree of interdependency that people experience determines the salient level of these perceptions.[6] This was determined by analyzing students' statements about self and other in different types of relationships. It was found that statements about intention, attitude, and emotion of self and other, were more frequent when the level of interdependency in a relationship was high rather than low. It thus appears that people understand one another and themselves better in a situation of intense mutuality and reciprocity.

With the advent of cultural sexuality, the concepts of "I" and "you" evolved with a fresh awareness of self and other, as well as an increased ability to empathize. At the most basic level the new sexual mutuality and interdependence overcame dominance relations between the sexes and promoted general egalitarian social interaction and communication. A major change in human behavior was occurring. It brought the earliest beginnings of modern humanity, transforming culture, social behavior, and the emotions.

The importance of human sexual behavior was noted by anthropologists Suggs and Marshall in 1971, a time when there was greater scholarship on the issue than now.[7] They said that cultural, sociological and emotional aspects of behavior which can be gathered under the term "sexual" are among the "most important of all facets of human existence." But they go on to note a strange paradox: despite its importance, the science of sexual behavior is not well developed. As a case in point, Dr. William Masters and Virginia Johnson were moved to begin their sexual study, published in 1966, because they discovered that female sexual anatomy was virtually medically unknown then.[8] In their investigation, Masters and Johnson did ground breaking work on women's sexuality, scientifically demonstrating the relationship between the female breast, the uterus, and female orgasm. Today it can still be said that the medical community does not fully comprehend, or is uninterested in female sexuality, particularly the erotic aspect of the female breasts and uterus, and this unawareness may have implications for diseases such as breast cancer and uterine cancer.

2

The family and the human pair-bond

AT THE START OF modern human culture, boundaries placed by nature on sexuality were broken. Humans no longer depended on the natural mating cycle, a cycle that in the chimpanzee confined sexual relations more or less to estrus, or monthly heat. Sex became highly voluntary, and reproduction and sexuality were separated. Because of the compelling experience of breast sex and deep intimacy and pleasure during copulation, women began to mate at any time in their menstrual cycle. Men therefore began to closely associate with them at all times, not just mainly around the time of female heat; men and women began to live together, mating regularly. Men became part of the family of women and children.

In cohabiting, men and women along with their children created the human family. Although today the family is described in myriad new ways, a basic description provided in 1949 by the well known sociologist, George Murdock, holds that a family is a social group that resides together, cooperates in economic matters, includes adults of both sexes at least two of whom have sexual relations, and functions to socialize the children.[1] Other sociologists have stressed the extended kinship aspect of the family. In considering the bi-parental family, the fact that the sexes, at some point in our pre-history, began to relate sexually as equals and to reside together is significant because it enabled the life sustaining cooperation and communication that are characteristic of humanity, and the concept of egalitarianism was introduced into human society.

The bi-parental family can be regarded as a source from which modern human culture emanates, but its beginnings are hidden in the depths of prehistory. In considering the family of some 200,000 to 100,000 years ago, the time of the rise of anatomically modern human beings, it is useful to make comparisons with our primate cousins, the chimpanzees, with whom we share a common ancestor and almost 99% of our genetic material. These close relatives in the animal kingdom do not share our life style. They are highly sexually promiscuous and their living arrangements are extremely different from ours. The chimpanzee family unit consists of a female and her offspring. The male progenitor does not provide food for them, and the young are nutritionally on their own after weaning at about five years of age, as described by Nancy Makepeace Tanner in her book, *On Becoming Human*.[2] In contrast, in the human situation, a shift occurred from promiscuity and exhibitionism (though still indulged in in our fantasies and in some lifestyles) to pair-bonding and private sex. A sexual revolution took place in the human past, whereby mated adults began to share an emotional bond and increased sexual pleasure, and to live together for varying lengths of time, even for a lifetime. Consequently, we began to feed one-another, and do the same for our children for many years past their time of weaning, that is, we began to work for one another.

The philosopher and social scientist, Frederick Engels, who wrote about sex and the family in *The Origin of the Family, Private Property and the State,* considered pairing to have existed from the earliest stages of humanity, acknowledging the role of cooperation and tolerance in the transition from the lower animals.[3] He noted that the first division of labor occurred between men and women for the propagation of children, each sex controlling the implements of their own work while living in communal, sharing households composed of kinship groups. Within this early social structure, the productivity of labor which provides the essentials of life, such as food, increasingly developed, resulting in a more complex society. As time went on, there ensued private property, differences in wealth, classes of people antagonistic to each other, and an end to what Engels considered to be the original supremacy of women.

Providing food for one's mate is a hallmark of the human pair bond, as signified by the act of bride and groom feeding wedding cake to each other. Bernard Chapais discusses cooperative provisioning and food sharing between pair-bonded mates in his book, *Primeval Kinship: How Pair Bonding Gave Birth to Human Society.*[4] But other mammals besides humans share food, for instance the dog; and mammals show affection for one another, as does the cat; and some, such as the prairie vole and the gibbon, are pair-bonded and monogamous, although infidelity is often observed. The human pair-bond is set apart from these other cases by the complex way that a man and woman are capable of relating to each other, with empathy, cooperation, tolerance, and advanced communication: we are often said to be in love.

Love is the emotion we associate with the human pair-bond. In his book, *Emotion Concepts,* Zoltan Kovecses, in discussing non-platonic love, says that in ideal cases the emotion of love requires sex as an antecedent.[5] Sexual intercourse does not always presuppose personal closeness and intimacy, but when sex is warm and intimate Kovecses refers to it as being closely associated with love. He says that affectionate, intimate sexual behavior is qualitatively different from mere copulation – that sex must be enriched to be thought of as loving. The change in the course of human evolution to the practice of sexual breast love was just such an enrichment, whereby mates were not merely copulating as required by nature. Instead they began to indulge in a new kind of milky generosity by the female, and extra attention by the male – a human cultural sexuality involving the breast, the organ of maternal love. In the process, reciprocal care ensued, and the emotional distance between the sexes was diminished.

Similar to Kovecses, the psychologist Robert Sternberg includes sex in his concept of love.[6] In his triangular love theory, love has three main components: passion, commitment, and intimacy. Passion is concerned with physical attraction and sexual consummation. Commitment arises with cognitive qualities that function to maintain love, such as the recognition of love or the decision to love. Intimacy refers to feelings of closeness, connectedness, and bondedness, accompanied by the desire to share and to help one another. We recognize this mingling of love and sex named by Sternberg as very human and qualitatively different from the sex of the chimpanzee. This suggests that at some point in time there was a move away from a mode of sex governed by nature – a transformation in the relationship between the sexes. Cultural breast sex became the precursor of love.

The mating system of our early human ancestors changed to one that creates a bond between mates, and there are many theories as to when and how this happened. It is claimed here that the key to the conversion was the female breast, the mammary gland for which our class, the mammals, is named. So basic is this organ that much weight can be given to the way it is used. To be specific, at some time in our prehistory females began to use the breast as an organ of sexuality during copulation, engendering increased pleasure, profound intimacy, mutual knowledge, empathy, cooperation, and love between the sexes. Furthermore this way of relating was passed on to succeeding generations. The sex researcher, Alfred Kinsey, in 1953 commented that the male mouth on the female breast is a sexual behavior that is particularly human, an observation noted by several authors in the field.[7] In drawing a contrast with other living creatures, Kinsey noted that among the lower mammals, stimulation of the female breast by males is relatively rare, but he found that manual and oral stimulation of women's breasts by men are techniques in marriage which are used on occasion by a large percentage of couples. I believe that woman, in her desire for sexual breast love, and man, in his acceptance of her desire, were accomplices in a new sort of biological and social relationship essential to the evolution of the pair-bond, marriage, and the family.

Pair-bonding is a basic phenomenon in human behavior, and it is linked to sexual activity as described by several authorities. Zoologist Desmond Morris maintained that "the naked ape is the sexiest primate alive," and he focused on the heightened sexuality of humanity as the foundation of the human pair-bond.[8] He is in accord with Kinsey in noting the behavioral attention that the adult human male devotes to the breasts of the female. Morris' concept is based on what he terms "improvements," over the other primates in sexual behavior, including the attainment of human female orgasm. What is significant about his thesis, I think, is his overall scheme, which proposes that the evolution of the fundamental human pair-bond is linked to enriched human sexuality.

The enhanced sex of humanity represents a shared experience of positive emotions. Because female desire for sexual breast love is facilitated by a partner, it invites satisfying the partner in return, strengthening the experience, and making the emotion of love possible between mates. The orgasm attained by each partner is cooperative, complex, and intense – engendering passion and commitment. With rewarding and reciprocal good feelings, a positive relationship with positive emotions can develop, reinforcing the pair-bond. Significantly, J. M. Gottman, who studied the dynamics of how people think and feel about each other, came to the conclusion that most marriages fail through a process of rising negative emotions.[9]

Cultural sexuality and the evolution of the family have far reaching implications. Even if humans are the unsurpassed sexual animal, our sexuality is nevertheless different from a raw, primitive, openly practiced sexuality. Along with the pair-bond and the formation of the human family there was a change away from the aggressive sex of our remote predecessors. Sex became hidden so as to diminish rivalry and jealous disruption. Humans developed a type of sexuality that models cooperation, not dominance – a more mutually rewarding form of sex that entails equality between the sexes, an incipient form of overall social egalitarianism.

The geneticist Theodosius Dobzhansky, author of *Mankind Evolving,* in noting the human reputation for being the sexiest animal, comments that at least humanity has made its "sexual urges less acutely competitive" than they were in our distant past.[10] He goes on to say that mates living together and cooperating made possible extended families and eventually other institutions, such as "clans, tribes, and nations," and that cooperation made "communication a necessity and stimulated the development of language." From this account we can extrapolate that much of who we are today depends on loving and less competitive sex. Starting with pair-bonding and the family, cultural social institutions depend on the kind of love characteristic of cultural sexuality, here identified as sexual breast love.

3

The breast and the love hormone

WE KNOW THAT BETWEEN mammalian mothers and their nursing infants there is a strong intimate bond, as described for chimpanzees by Jane Goodall in her book, *The Chimpanzees of Gombe*.[1] For instance consider the affection that is shared between a nursing chimpanzee mother and her offspring. So deep is the bond that a three year old chimpanzee infant will often not survive if its mother dies, even though it is fairly self sufficient at that age. And a chimpanzee mother will carry a dead infant around while grieving for days. In contrast there is no strong bond between the mating adult male and female chimpanzee; according to Goodall chimps walk away after copulation without either male or female being emotionally moved. Comparing this behavior described by Goodall with our own, it can be said that at some time in human experience, intimacy of the type found between mother and infant became possible between adult female and adult male, resulting in love between the sexes, and bringing with it the rising of *Homo sapiens*, that is, ourselves.

The idea that the breast is an erotic organ, whether suckled by an infant or by a mate, still elicits shame even in scientific discourse today. Consider the anthropologist, Robin Fox's statement: "Suckling responses in the mother are strongly sexual, as we now know and can admit."[2] There is always hesitancy to admit the erotic nature of suckling. The feminist and sociologist, Alice Rossi, was an expert on this taboo subject.[3] She was one of the few social scientists to analyze the erotic nature of the emotional bond between mother and infant. Rossi notes the close connection between maternalism and sexuality in mammalian females, and she says that Western society has not dealt with this link. She illuminates the connection by describing the biological hormone, oxytocin, which increases in the female body with suckling at the breast during nursing. She goes on to say that oxytocin is also well known to be associated with the rhythmic, pleasurable uterine contractions of orgasm, as well as with the strong and sharp uterine contractions of childbirth. Of interest, oxytocin release in the body occurs with orgasm in both men and women.

The hormone closely associated with both breastfeeding and sexuality, is oxytocin, as determined by biologists studying its effects in the human body. The following is a short catalogue of discoveries about oxytocin, which is found in the blood and brain of both sexes. In women it is a powerful uterotonic agent that causes contractions of the uterus during childbirth,[4] and it is associated with the prevention of postpartum hemorrhage.[5] It was shown by Irons in 1994 that with nipple stimulation, that blood loss tended to be reduced in the third stage of labor when the placenta is delivered, and it was felt that a larger study was warranted.[6] With nipple stimulation during breastfeeding oxytocin is released into the blood and it is active in milk ejection, as determined by McNeely in 1983.[7] Carmichael documented in 1987 that levels of circulating oxytocin increased during sexual stimulation and arousal, with a peak during orgasm in both women and men.[8] Blaicher, 1999, found that oxytocin plays a role in sexual arousal in women and it was thought that this was a response to stimulation of the areola surrounding the nipple and stimulation of the genital tract.[9]

As determined by Amico and Finley in 1986, blood oxytocin was significantly increased above baseline in response to breast stimulation in two of five women during their normal menstrual cycle.[10] Both tactile and mechanical pump stimulation were intermittently used. In 18 of 19 pregnant women in the Amico and Finley study, mean oxytocin was significantly higher after nipple stimulation than before. In one non-postpartum woman who induced lactation for the purpose of breast feeding her adopted infant, oxytocin increased during tactile and mechanical pump stimulation of the breast as well as during suckling.

Leake, in 1984, determined that with mechanical pump stimulation of the nipples, oxytocin increases in the blood during the luteal phase of the menstrual cycle, but no increase was seen in the follicular phase of the cycle.[11] Salonia and others working in 2005 showed that blood plasma oxytocin is significantly lower during the luteal phase of the menstrual cycle compared with both the follicular and ovulatory phases.[12] Of special interest in thinking about breast sex, it was found by Auerbach and Avery in 1981 that nipple stimulation in women without prior pregnancy induces milk secretion in small amounts.[13]

Animal studies have been the basis for research into brain oxytocin. In prairie voles, brain oxytocin is important for pair-bonding induced by mating, especially in females, as shown by Neumann in 2008, and he also found that it reduces stress in male rats.[14] Witt and Insell determined in 1991 that brain oxytocin is essential for the regulation of sexual behavior in female rats;[15] and according to Kendrick, 1991, both brain and blood oxytocin are instrumental in the uterine contractions of sheep during birth.[16] Importantly, Neumann indicates that in humans, brain oxytocin exerts similar effects to those shown in animal studies.

The area of the brain that is responsive to oxytocin, promotes both nurturance behavior and partner preference or bonding, and interestingly it is also involved in female sexual receptivity, according to Panksepp.[17] He says that in the female brain, areas responsible for nurturance and social bonding may have arisen from neural circuits responsible for female sexual function. He also notes that brain oxytocin facilitates nurturance in the male, and a surge of brain oxytocin occurs with ejaculation, again indicating a relationship between nurturance and sexual function.

From the foregoing it is clear why oxytocin is sometimes referred to as the love hormone. It is associated with nipple excitation, lovemaking, orgasm, contractions of the uterus, milk release to the nursing infant, and it reduces stress, making us feel good. Of special interest, oxytocin promotes pair-bonding. While in mammals the pair-bond is intrinsic to the mother-offspring nursing pair, humans can construct an additional pair-bond, a cultural love bond between adult mates. In this liaison, the breasts and oxytocin are participants via the erotic use of the breasts in adult lovemaking. You might say that "cultural" oxytocin was introduced into human life.

4

Breast eroticism and the uterine connection

FOR WOMEN, THE EXTREME pleasure of sex occurs when the uterus contracts, which can be facilitated and heightened via the breasts. In a ground breaking work in 1966, the sexual interconnection between the breasts and the uterus was described by Masters and Johnson.[1] Not only did they record the pulsating of the uterus during female orgasm, they also demonstrated a relationship between stimulated breasts and female orgasm. This look at the eroticism of the uterus and its corollary, the eroticism of the breasts, carried out by Master's and Johnson was exceptional because the study of human sexuality did not progress far beyond their work. Despite their observation that research into human sexuality was then in its infancy, this difficult topic was subsequently all but abandoned by the scientific community. We should be grateful to Master's and Johnson for giving us all that they did. The women and men in their inquiry were chosen for their ability to attain orgasm (sometimes termed a bias of the study), and the study's descriptions indicated that women used breast stimulation as an aid in reaching their climaxes. Masters and Johnson reported that the uterus contracts during orgasm, and of particular interest here, they noted that woman's orgasm could be reached with breast stimulation alone.

As we have seen, breast eroticism has a physiological tie to uterine eroticism, and women's appreciation of the intense good feelings that result from taking advantage of this link must have preceded the adoption of widespread breast sex. It could be said that ancestral women made a practical discovery about their own bodies, a technological finding at the working level, leading to innovative behavior. This idea fits well with the viewpoint of Marcel Mauss concerning the body, although it would better suit present purposes to substitute the word "humanity" for his word "man".[2] Mauss thought that the body was a "natural instrument". He referred to it as "man's first and most natural technical object, and at the same time technical means." Exactly how woman began to appreciate the sexual capability of her breasts is not known. This physiological knowledge might have accumulated gradually at first, the practice slowly passing from person to person through observation and imitation, and then suddenly in an overwhelming way the method caught on. One outcome of the new understanding and practice was an improvement in reproduction. With breast sex and the subsequent bonding between men and women, joint participation in child-raising became possible: people were able to provide superior care for each child. This reproductive advantage would have hastened the spread of cultural sexuality.

As we learned from Dr. Paré, infant breast feeding has a pleasurable link to the uterus—a hushed up connection and somewhat difficult topic. The psychoanalyst, Jonathan Slavin, recounts the experience of a patient who felt deep love for her infant son, and who was concerned about her emotions.[3] She was anxious about the erotic feelings activated when she breast-fed her baby, although she knew that this can be a typical experience among nursing mothers.

Turning again to Alice Rossi who is very astute on this issue, she notes that the connection between sexuality and maternalism makes "evolutionary" sense: that with the erotogenic good feelings of breastfeeding a mother is more likely to nurse her baby longer, and the uterus quickly returns to its pre-pregnancy condition.[4] She comments on the hormone oxytocin which is released from the posterior pituitary gland in the brain with sexual intercourse and during nursing. She names oxytocin as a clear link between sexuality and maternalism because it is associated with the uterine contractions of orgasm that aid the sperm in reaching the oviduct where it meets the egg, and also with the contractions of childbirth. She identifies oxytocin with nipple erection during either "nursing or love-play," that is, "whether the sucking is by an infant or a lover."

The difference for a woman between her love for her infant versus for her lover, is that breast-feeding an infant and breast sex have different functions: one to nourish; the other to have sex. Both acts have eroticism at the core, but in the case of infant feeding, the mother's genitals are not involved, so infant breast love is pleasurable but not sexual. With breast sex, the genitals of the adult mates are involved, so the eroticism becomes sexual.

Alice Rossi, citing nipple erection during love-play and its association with oxytocin, provides a biosocial perspective on cultural sexuality. Masters and Johnson who describe the use of the breasts during sexual activity present scientific evidence for the efficacy of breast sex in attaining woman's orgasm. Much research remains to be done in this nascent area but it is clear that our biology and culture are intimately intertwined. This is in keeping with the main thesis of this book that the use of the breast for sexual purposes is the epitome of cultural sexuality, occurring at the nexus of biology and modern human culture, a long sought intersection.

5

The change to the family and the sharing of love

THE CHANGE TO LOVE and the family brought with it the problems and the potential conflicts of close family living. If humans are indeed pre-eminently sexual creatures, then this may be reflected in various interpersonal relationships, including in family relationships. There are many ways that this can play out. On the one hand, strong feelings within the family can be quite innocent and ordinary, just as a mother's deep love for her nursing infant is innocent and ordinary. However, when love must be shared, then conflicted feelings may result, with possible disruptions to the family.

How do these conflicts and tensions arise in the family? A lot has to do with the pair-bond and the close family unit within which both parents are potential care givers. The anthropologist and psychologist, Melford Spiro, known for his emphasis on the universal in human culture, develops the idea of factors in the human family everywhere that lead to tensions.[1] The children feel great affection for their parents, who are the ones who gratify their needs. However, since there is a sexual relationship between the parents, the children must share their mother's love and affection with their father. Therefore parents also frustrate their children's needs. With the arrival of a new infant, the love must be further shared and sibling rivalry can appear. In the case of non-human mammals, with the birth of a sibling, the older offspring's feeding relationship with the mother is terminated, but not in the case of human children whose dependence on parents is typically very prolonged. This situation provides a lot of time for various emotions to develop between dyads, or pairs, within the family. Spiro comments that: "so far as their emotional texture is concerned, we would expect that in any society the relationships among all of the dyads comprising the family would be characterized by strong ambivalence, and that children would develop both an Oedipus complex and sibling rivalry."

The anthropologist L.L. Langness comments on the nature of the Oedipus complex.[2] He says that the maintenance of the family is of paramount importance to its participants, but complex relationships within the family have the potential not only to maintain it but to destroy it. In the latter case, strong emotions in the family can result in the condition known as the Oedipus complex, an unconscious feeling in the son of strong love for his mother and jealousy toward his father. There is a corresponding complex associated with the daughter. The Oedipus complex does not result from biology, according to Langness, but from child raising requirements within the family. However, the pair-bond that enables love and the formation of the human family is also instrumental in quelling incestuous feelings that arise there; faced with their parents' strong relationship, children are encouraged to seek sex elsewhere.

Some cultures institute an incest taboo, known in preliterate societies, to strengthen the pair-bond and to preventing sibling mating. Establishment of the incest taboo was eventually accompanied by the introduction of rules of marriage and kinship, forbidding marriage between certain pairs of close relatives. These rules were often complex, for instance, allowing marriage between some cousins but not between others. Regarding incest and siblings, rather than being sexually attracted to one another, it was claimed by the sociologist Edvard Westermarck that children who are raised together before the age of six, become sexually desensitized to one another in a natural way and are less likely to marry later.[3] His theory has been promoted by some authorities, and criticized by others. Sibling rivalry, a well known family phenomenon, would also seem to work against sibling mating, even if attractions exist. However, in cultures such as in ancient Egypt, and in Hawaii, sibling mating and marriage were permissible and served to maintain family dynasties of the rulers.

Parents who are secure in their relationship are able to respond with understanding to the developing sexuality of their children. Returning to the ideas of Jonathan Slavin, who analyzes the feeling of love within the family: the affection that develops between members of a family always has an element of sexual attraction. This is because, he says, when individuals are alone together for long periods of time, as happens in family living, sexual feelings for one another develop. Not only do children have these attractions to their parents, parents have sexual feelings for their children. According to Slavin, there is a need to accept what he terms, "ordinary, normal sexuality between parents and children that spans the entire development process."[4] In discussing benign ways to address this situation and help the child, he notes that: "the parent's responsiveness to the child's developing sexual interest is crucial for the normal integration of the self as a loving, lovable, and sexual person."[5] He calls this responsiveness, an "innocent" kind of sexual relating.

The concept of innocent sexuality between parents and children can be found in several cultures, along with practices that, although not subtle, are appropriate to the culture. Evidence gathered in two diverse societies illustrates this. For instance the children of the Copper Inuit of north central Canada are known to observe their parents in lovemaking, and parents tease their children about their intimate parts from the earliest years; these Inuit also allow childhood sex games in which parent behavior is imitated, as observed by Raymond DeCoccola.[6] The Saramaka of Suriname, South America have similar customs in which the grandparents touch children's genitals in a teasing manner, and three and four year olds play at sexual intercourse, as related by Sally Price.[7] They are continually reminded of their sex from infancy. In these ways human sexuality is acknowledged and taught within the family or community, with no guilt attached.

6

Incest in past human society

THE ARGUMENT OF THIS book is that the adoption of breast sexuality was a pivotal behavior, enabling the cooperative lifestyle of *Homo sapiens.* Some understanding of early modern human lifestyle can be gained by studying extant preliterate groups. The ways of today's surviving hunter-gatherer societies are generally thought to provide indirect information about the lifestyle of earlier such societies. In this regard, anthropologists studying contemporary pre-literate societies have documented, in the ethnographic record, the sexual use of the breast and its variations. As has been suggested, when breast sexuality was discovered its practice was maintained and spread; the change to this cultural style of sexuality and bonding between men and women was voluntary. Knowledge of it was transmitted from generation to generation.

Interestingly, its discovery during the course of human experience may have been related to incest. One might imagine a time and locale of isolation and hardship for ancestral females and their offspring, not unlike the background described in some human origin stories. At this transitional time in human development, with adversity extending over some period of time, and a possible earlier onset of adolescence than today, prolonged breastfeeding may have been necessary, and it allowed an opportunity for breast sex to happen. Studies of various human societies throughout the world show that, on occasion, women breastfeed their children, even today, into the child's adolescent years. This is the case, for instance among the Lepchas of Sikkim, according to Gorer and Hutton.[1] From the past, a temple wall of ancient Egypt depicts the deity Isis nursing her son Horus as an adolescent, indicating an ancient custom.[2] See Figure 1.

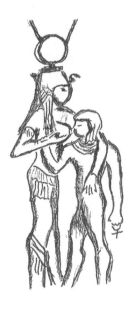

Figure 1
Isis suckling her son, Horus, as a youth; c. 30 BCE – CE 14. Outer wall of Temple of Hathor, Denderah. Drawing by the author from a photo in Anne Baring and Jules Cashford, *Myth of the Goddess: Evolution of an Image.*

Incest may have been an important though transient practice in transitional *Homo sapiens* life. Sigmund Freud, in his book *Totem and Taboo*, claimed that opposition to incest played a role in the development of humanity, and for many pre-literate human societies there are prominent incest taboos, suggesting the former potency of the practice.[3] But according to the anthropologist, Robin Fox not all incest taboos are equally strong; it all depends on the society.[4] The sexual behavior of our human line at some point in time several hundred thousand years ago was no doubt distinctive, differing from today's sexual behavior, and incest may have fleetingly been practiced among early modern humans. Interestingly incest is not a common occurrence among the chimpanzees, according to Jane Goodall, and the reason for this is not really known.[5] One possibility is the character of weaning.

There is roughness and finality in chimpanzee weaning, during which the mother definitively severs her intimate breastfeeding relationship with her offspring at age four or five years. In another primate, the rhesus monkey, explicit breast eroticism has been recorded—identified as autoerotic in nature by the primatologist, C. R. Carpenter.[6] Female rhesus monkeys have been observed to suck on or pull at their own breasts when they are most fertile, the time of their greatest sexual activity. Similar autoerotic behavior has not been reported for chimpanzees, but breastfeeding has an erotic component and forceful weaning terminates the sensual sensations of breastfeeding and the intimate relationship with offspring in preparation for further reproductive activity of the mother chimp.

As in chimpanzee life, incest may not have been a common occurrence among the very earliest members of the human line, only making a brief appearance. Along with cultural sexuality, incest may have occurred in early bi-parental family living attempts, which included for the first time both the adult female and male, and children, who remained in the family past adolescence. If incest did occupy a place in the early beginnings of modern humanity, it was subsequently forbidden because of its power to cause conflict. Incest is not the norm in human society and not typical of human behavior today.

The idea that original incest was important has a basis in folk accounts of the origin of humanity. For instance, the ancient folklore of the Inuit tells of isolated mothers and sons, far from any other human company, in which the sons become the husbands. The narrative and associated song are published in the book *Northern Voices,* edited by Penny Petrone, a collection of writings and oral memories of the Inuit people.[7] This is the story of two women who were described as dangerous. When their husbands, who were brothers, were murdered, sex was forced on the women. In retaliation, they made "water" in the mouth of one man, and smothered him. The story recounts how the two women, with the mother of the murdered brothers, fled from the scene, going across the ice to escape. They were ultimately stranded with their babies on a frozen island, now known as the island of Southampton. Such stories were popularly regarded as historical accounts according to Petrone. After a while the women lay with their own boys, whose growth became so stunted that the women continued to carry them in the deep amauts or hoods of their parkas. From this protected place, the husbands instructed the women in the ways of hunting walrus and seal. A shaman, representing the pinnacle of old Inuit culture as both physician and priest, having found them out, attempted to kill them, but the women, being shamans themselves, sang a magic song expressing their strong love for their small mates, and they and their husbands prevailed. This creation story was told to Rasmussen by Naukatjik, an Iglulik.

> *My husband I carry in my amaut,*
> *Love him and kiss him,*
> *And hide him away now,*
> *Because he is hunted by one*
> *Who is not a real human being.*
> *My husband I carry in my amaut,*
> *Love him and kiss him.*
> *Ajaja – ajaja*
>
> *Walrus I hunt*
> *With my husband in the amaut,*
> *Following his wise counsel,*
> *Loving him and kissing him,*
> *And hiding him now*
> *That he is hunted by one*
> *Who is not a real human being,*

A shaman that seeks to kill him.
Ajaja –ajaja (Petrone, p11)

Not only folk accounts, but ancient religions reflect the remote past of human experience. In contemplating the possible incestuous origins of humanity, we can look back to around 3000 BCE at the Mesopotamian religions of the Bronze Age. Anne Baring and Jules Cashford have written extensively about the subject.[8] The Sumerians of the Bronze Age were the inventors of writing, and as described in their poetry, they worshipped a goddess of sex and love, whose husband was also her son, or in some versions, her brother. These were the deities Inanna and Dumuzi. At about the same time in Babylon there was a similar pair, known as Ishtar and her son-lover, Tamuz meaning "Faithful Son". It was thought that the passionate relationship of the goddess with her husband brought sacred love to the world.

Sumerian poetry celebrates the exploits of Inanna. Significantly, she is said to have made an epic journey by boat to bring back the special properties of civilization to her city, Uruk, including the gifts of wisdom, understanding, and awareness of sexual intercourse. The acquisition of knowledge and a new comprehension of sexuality is a theme in other creation myths as well—those of Ethiopian, Hebrew/ Christian, and Inuit origin, where incest is also a factor.

Another of Inanna's voyages took her through the perils of the underworld, and having successfully returned, she sent her son/ husband, Dumuzi, the god of growing things, to take her place below. Together they brought about the change of the seasons. Fertility was thought to be suspended for the part of the year that Dumuzi was gone. When he returned to earth the couple mated, causing celebration among the people with rites of rebirth and regeneration. According to Baring and Cashford, similar religions were found all over the Near East and the Mediterranean area, for instance the worship of the Egyptian goddess Isis and her brother-lover Osiris. So pervasive was the worship of Isis that the kings of Egypt had themselves depicted as her sons.

The breast, both nourishing and sexual, appears in stories of the Egyptian Isis. It was believed that the lap of the goddess represented the throne of Egypt and that a king who ascended the throne received nourishment by suckling the breast of Isis, affirming his right to rule. In a painting from about 1300 BCE, Isis is shown putting her nipple to the mouth of King Seti I of the Nineteenth Dynasty. Scholars of ancient religions, Baring and Cashford, in their book mentioned above, comment on Isis and King Seti: "She nurses him from her breast, giving the term 'son-lover of the goddess' an unusually precise image."[9]

Sexuality of the breast is with us still, perhaps suggestive of an incestuous ancestry, or at least of a return to scenes of infancy. In using the organ of maternity for adult erotic purposes, breast sex recalls the mother/infant relationship and thus may hint at incest and its taboo dimensions. The ethnographer, Bronislaw Malinowski in his account of life in the Trobriand Islands of the South Pacific, acknowledged the similar sensuous bodily contact inherent in both love-making and mothering.[10] In remarking on the naked clinging, and use of the breast for both the adult sexual act and for infant nutrition, he states: "The analogy between the preparatory actions of the sexual drive and the consummatory actions of the infantile impulse are remarkable." Another parallel between the two behaviors, nursing and the cultural sex act, is the power of the breast, both maternally and sexually, to foster the positive emotional bond of love.

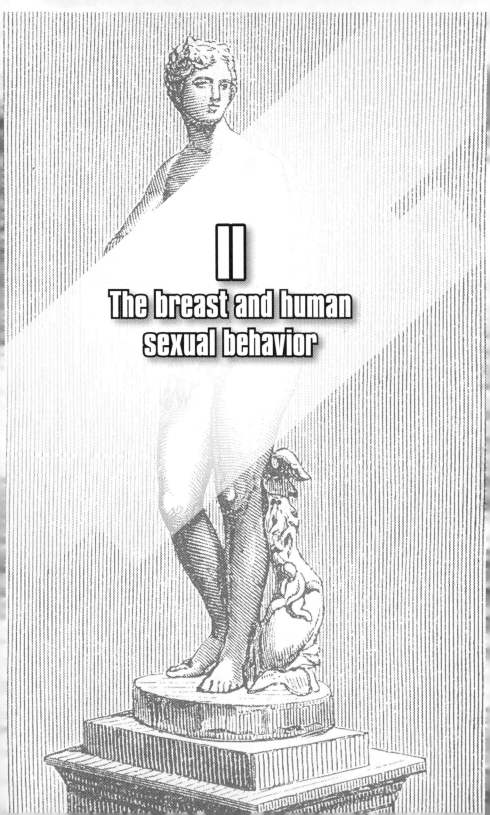

II
The breast and human sexual behavior

1

The journey of the breast

WHAT FOLLOWS IN CHAPTERS II, III, and IV are anthropological and other data suggesting that breast sex as a means of attaining female sexual pleasure and orgasm, is practiced world wide. Human invention of this sexual technique significantly distinguished the human sex act from that of other animals in a manner that was subsequently promoted by human culture. We will look at the cross-cultural evidence showing that woman's sexuality is associated with the breasts.

In the area of present-day reporting from the United States, Shere Hite's collection of women's testimony about their bodies and lives in The *Hite Report*, confirms that the breasts are here and now organs of eroticism.[1] The book, first published in 1976, and again in 2004, for the most part focuses on aspects of women's sexuality that have to do with the clitoris. However, many excerpts from the *Hite Report* demonstrate that contemporary women have sensual breasts and that they use their breasts as a means to obtain climax during intercourse and masturbation. Also in the realm of contemporary life in the U.S., the book *Women Speak about Their Breasts and Their*

Lives by Ayalah and Weinstock, highlights the sexuality of women's breasts, although at least one woman interviewed by the authors states that her breasts are not sexual.[2]

The intent in presenting the following accounts is to show that the female breast has been associated with the everyday sex of human beings everywhere. An opportunity to look at descriptions of various cultures from around the world is provided by the Human Relations Area Files, started by the anthropologist George Peter Murdock and maintained by Yale University. The files contain accounts of various cultures of the world from books published mostly in the early and mid-twentieth century with additional recent accounts. There is some focus on tribal cultures, which in many cases refer back to ancient, preliterate ways, allowing us to appreciate that breast sex is an ancestral practice. For the most part, the authors are anthropologists, sociologists, and linguists, who study and record the ways of diverse ethnic groups.

Excluded from this collection are the many unstudied cultures of the world that have disappeared, or that have never been observed. Also excluded is sexual knowledge acquired in the field by anthropologists and then suppressed due to a sense of taboo. Referring to worries by investigators that they might appear too interested in sex, Robert Suggs and Donald Marshall, in their book *Human Sexual Behavior,* conjectured that some sexual information remains forever in the heads of ethnographers rather than reported.[3] Where reporting does exist, as in the following qualitative descriptions from societies in vastly disparate areas of the world, it is seen that breast sex is a wide cultural phenomenon.

In *Sex and Repression in Savage Society,* Bronislaw Malinowski's implication is that, for a man, a revisit to infancy is suggested by the male actions in the sex act: his lips placed on the female nipple.[4] This might mean that one reason a man makes contact with a woman's breast is because he remembers the pleasant sensations of early closeness to his mother. What is just as likely is that he discovers the seductive power that the nipple has for a woman. In this case, the breasts epitomize both ripened femaleness and the female readiness to have sex.

As the ethnographic record shows, touching a woman's breasts can be a means of courting her, or of soliciting sex from her. The woman herself solicits sex by offering her breasts. In many cultures, with the development of her breasts, a young woman begins her sex life. Before that, she is considered not ready. With the advent of cultural sexuality, men and women for the first time became capable of being lovers, and in their quest for sexual orgasm, lovers began to assist each other. The interaction of male and female often has a ritual character to ensure the pleasure of both, and that helps the act come to fruition for both—usually woman first and then man. The cooperation of the male and female in the sexuality of the breast is shown in the ethnographic record, and is central to mutual pleasure, love, and intense interaction – the qualities of cultural sexuality.

In the U.S., much is made of men's obsession with women's breasts. Women themselves are obsessed with their breasts and the admiration they can bring, while at the same time perhaps not understanding their sexual potential. Many women, especially young women, are not knowledgeable about their bodies. Some women do the unthinkable: fill their breasts with silicon for alleged beautification and greater appeal, a procedure known to dull the feeling in the nipple. Before resorting to surgery, women should be able to be informed about their potentially erotic breasts by relevant books – essentially nonexistent today, even in sex education classes. This is admittedly a sensitive topic, but on the other hand, the lack of discourse on breast eroticism may contribute to sexual dysfunction and even to the high incidence of breast cancer. Women of simpler societies than that of the present day U.S, appear to have been more informed about the sexual potential of their breasts. The ways of these societies are fast disappearing and in many cases have been disapproved of, especially by missionaries. The ancient life-ways need to be re-examined for the insights they can bring.

Use of the female breast has been basic to our human style of sex throughout much of the world, but perhaps not so much in the

U.S. today. An anthropologist informed me that most humans do not use their breasts with sexual intent. It's not clear whom she had in mind. For women in the U.S., it may be that many do not rely on their breasts for sexual pleasure. There is certainly in the U.S. little openness or information on the topic of mammary sexuality, and women may be reluctant to enjoy an experience they perceive as not the norm. In contrast, in a YouTube video, *Who Owns the Breast: Street Talk Naija*, one may witness and listen to a discussion of breast sex and who enjoys it more, recorded on a city street in Nigeria, perhaps Lagos.[5]

Why is there so little recognition of breast sex in current discourse? The myth of Dracula, and similar satanic types, who suck blood and other bodily fluids, perhaps gives us a clue – a reference to unholy practices that have the power to turn people into animals. The tabooed nature of women's carnality is undeniable and may prompt women's refusal to speak of the erotic nature of their breasts. A concern of this book is: how do women feel about their breasts? One answer can be found in the conversation from Nigeria, referred to above, about "who owns the breast" and "why do men suck." In the dialogue between several people, we learn from a male conversant that if a woman didn't enjoy it so much, she wouldn't press the man's head closer to her breast. We learn from a female conversant that the reason a woman does this is that she wants it "more" and that she loves it.

Words such as these, women's words on breast sex, are hard to find, although we can "hear" women in the U.S. speak about these matters in *The Hite Report* by Shere Hite, noted at the beginning of this chapter. In the *Hite Report*, based on anonymous answers to a large, many faceted questionnaire, 48 women comment on their use of the breast during masturbation. One woman says: "I hardly ever come without simultaneous nipple stimulation."[6] In the same text, twelve women comment on breast use during intercourse. One gives a detailed description of intercourse, saying: "At the same time he plays with my nipples."[7] Also reported are instances of lesbian sexual breast contact.[8] The book is a good source of candid talk about sex, similar to a women's consciousness raising session, in which the important thing is not statistics but what is said.

Not only in Nigeria, and in the U.S., but in many cultures, the sexual role of the female breast can be discerned in its various aspects. Breast sex is evident in sexual playing, in joking, in both male and female solicitation of sex, in erotic desire, in seduction, in dance, in poetry and song, in myth, in courtship, in marriage, in foreplay, during intercourse, and in kinship and outside relationships. With a modicum of searching, the ethnographic record reveals the secrets of a taboo subject that is relevant to everyday lives everywhere. It indicates how basically alike we all are in matters of cultural sexuality, no matter where we live: Asia, North America, Europe, Oceania, South America or other areas of our Earth.

2

The breast in the sex life of young people – sexual desire

IN MANY CULTURES, YOUNG people desiring to have sex attend community dances arranged for that purpose. In the early 20th century, Cora DuBois visited Alor, an Indonesian island of the Lesser Sunda islands which include Bali, and in 1944 she reported on aspects of culture on that island including sexuality.[1] According to DuBois, much erogenous feeling centers on women's breasts. At dances and when playing around, if young people are away from their elders, young men solicit intercourse of young women by touching their breasts. In describing how his hands and the hands of other males in these situations move about at random and touch girls breasts, one youth explained to DuBois that touching a girl's breast causes her "spirit to fly away" and she is compelled to sleep with a man. In one form or other, this is a basic and durable idea among various cultures, attesting to the power of a woman's breasts to arouse desire and sexual passion in her. One of DuBois' informants told the story of a young woman's desire and how she expressed it. The woman kept coming up to dance with him all night, and at one point as they moved into the shadows, she placed the man's hand on her breast. He played with her breast and he would have had intercourse with her he said, if there had not been a bright moon. He claimed that toward dawn he saw her go off to sleep with another man who had fondled her breasts because she had to sleep with someone after that. According to DuBois, a common euphemism for having intercourse is "pulling the breasts," since it is assumed that no woman can help being excited by such a caress, or would be able to resist a man who approached her like that.

Seduction by touching the breast, as described in Alor, is also found in other societies in the context of a dance or other social gathering. Bronoslaw Malinowski tells the story of the *karibom,* a slow rhythmic social promenade that takes place in the Trobriand Islands off the east coast of Papua New Guinea.[2] Many people take part in the walk, from grandparents with grandchildren, to women with babies, and pairs of lovers. Because the *karibom* takes place on dark moonless evenings, it provides an opportunity for erotic approach, more so than at ordinary dances. Malinowski notes that there are a number of ways of erotic approach which can be carried out during the *karibom* by a boy who is walking in back of the girl he is interested in: one way is that from this place he can touch her breasts, an act which the natives of these islands say is effective in stimulating her erotic interest.

For the young people of the Gusii tribe of Kenya, marriage ceremonies furnish a venue to meet each other. According to Robert Alan LeVine, these ceremonies are one of the few places for premarital contact.[3] Young men accompany the groom to the bride's house where they can dance with girls. Unsupervised dancing goes on for a good part of the night and afterward young men and women sleep in the same house. Kissing and fondling of breasts takes place, and these intimacies at marriage dances often result in sexual intercourse, although participants may claim that chastity was maintained.

Among the tribal Santals of West Bengal, India, and Bangladesh, the breasts have a great appeal at dances when the two sexes mingle closely and join hands. The sight of the breasts at a dance induces sexual attraction and may lead to intimacy. Charulal Mukherjea tells us that as the dance progresses, there is talk of love; the man warms up and seeks a response from his partner – he presses her wrists in a nonchalant manner, and if she presses in return, the man will frequently touch and press her breast with his elbow, for instance.[4] With the touching of the young woman's breast, the sexual understanding is complete, and the couple excuse themselves and retire to a private spot away from the party.

The allure of the breasts according to Mukherjea is the subject of many Santal folk songs. In a verse in his book, *The Santals,* one of several verses that illustrate breast eroticism, a young man sings to a young woman that her body reminds him of ripe mangos, and he pictures her breasts as bel-fruits.[5] He asks her to whom her body and breasts belong, and to whom they will bring pleasure. She replies that he shouldn't worry or "weep", because they are hers but are "meant" for him. Reciprocally, she asks him who has access to his loincloth, and he answers that she too should not worry, because they both do.

W. G. Archer collected and commented on hundreds of Santal songs in the mid- twentieth century. This folk song appears in his 1974 book, *The Hill of Flutes.*[6]

> *Under the bushes*
> *Which two are struggling?*
> *The girl has caught his chest*
> *The boy is holding her breasts*
> *Boy and girl they rock together.*
>
> *Under a bush they are struggling*
> *For a bun of hair*
> *The girl is saying*
> *'I will hold your belt*
> *and never leave it'*

The boy is saying
'I will live
Holding your breasts.' (124)

In the following song, a young man identifies a woman's breasts as having induced his love. The woman signifies her sexual desire by asking her potential lover to take her breasts in his hands. The song appears in W. G. Archer.[7]

Girl: *Boy, I am now a mother. And you are still untried. What is it roused your love?*

Boy: *Your thighs are mangoes. Your breasts are the half-ripe fruits of a bel. I saw them and they fired my love.*

Girl: *Where are you from, boy? Where are you going? What is your village? My body is a mango. My breasts are golden marrows. Lift and take them in your hands.* (111)

A story of premarital sexual desire among the Navaho Indians of North America is told by Walter Dyk, written with his Navaho consultant, Left Handed.[8] Although the preliminaries in this account are similar to the previous examples of young sex, the ending is different. A young man and woman are putting sheep in the corral, and in the evening when the job is almost done, the woman begins to tickle the young man and to touch him all over. He responds by touching her breasts. He holds her breasts and touches her between the legs and she gets down on the ground. But since the young man is inexperienced, he does no more than touch her. The author says in his narration that although he knows she likes being fondled and wants to have sex, after much fooling around the boy ends up returning to his mother's Hogan; such is often the sex life of young people – one of frustration or self doubt.

Hesitancy is more typically exhibited by the woman rather than the man, as in the following folk story from the Cuna, a Caribbean tribe living in Panama, Central America. The story appears in an account of premarital sex among the Cuna by Nils Magnus Holmer.[9]

It is the tale of Sususappin and his love for Turtle Woman's daughter. The young man is brought by the girl's mother to the sleeping loft to court her daughter there. He asks the girl's permission to feel her genitals, and when she hesitates, he asks again. At both these requests the girl descends the ladder and asks her mother if Sususappin is acting strangely. Her mother reassures her that this is the usual way that men behave in courtship. Finally Sususappin asks if he can feel her breasts. Now he apparently has found the right way to woo her, for she allows him to feel her breasts. The two appear to be satisfied, her breasts having played a featured role in the courtship.

The men of the Jivaro natives of Ecuador have a custom of courting women with a preparation called semica that is supposed to aid in the prospects for success in love, according to Matthew Williams Stirling.[10] The suitor first goes to the forest and collects and grinds certain leaves and mixes them with a sweet smelling herb and grease; or he may buy it. Then he carries the semica in a bamboo tube to the house of his intended, and in the course of visiting her he arranges to rub the mixture on the palms of her hands and on her breasts. If she accepts his gift of semica and his attention to her breasts, it indicates that she returns his affection.

Love is not always reciprocated, sometimes prompting the rejected one to write ironic poetry, as in the following pessimistic verses from the Amhara people of Ethiopia. This poem about a love liaison gone wrong employs an image that refers to the sexual breast. The poem was collected by Donald Nathan Levine.[11]

> *Fish on the cliff, baboons in the sea;*
> *The ass after honey, while hay draws the bee;*
> *On a baking-pan of wax, butter to see;*
> *Or a monk from Zegamel monastery*
> *In the pagan land of Metcha to bury;*
> *With an unsuited person in love to be;*
> *Thus has it ended, my affair with thee.*
> *Leave it, forget it, just let it rest –*
> *A hapless ass at a hyena's breast.* (270)

3

Prohibitions against touching the breasts in courtship

THE BELIEF THAT FONDLING a woman's breasts is seductive, and that, if done skillfully in a dark corner at a dance, it will induce the woman to have sexual intercourse, was strongly expressed by the Santals, the Alorese, and the Trobriand Islanders. But if the culture does not approve of premarital sex, such petting is potentially dangerous for an inexperienced girl to submit to. For Italian American girls, up until perhaps the 1950s, such overtures had to be repulsed in order for the girl to maintain her honor. This is described by Robert Orsi in his depiction of a "dangerous" dance in Italian Harlem.[1] There the boys expected their advances to be resisted, and one boy was reported to have commented on the decency of a particular girl because she had given him a hard slap when he spoke of her beautiful breasts. Orsi points out that the girl's behavior was known as "managing one's boyfriend."

For the Kapaukans of West New Guinea fondling of the breasts is not supposed to happen at young peoples' dances. The dances are held for the purpose of formally arranging dates and marriages, but they can also serve as places to informally flirt with the opposite sex. Often things get out of control, with he boys provocatively standing in the way of the girls, leading to pushing and shoving; and the girls, for their part, take hair decorations from the boys' heads, which are then snatched back. This scene is described by Leopold Pospisil, who did field work there.[2] All seems to be in playful good fun until the small torches of fire that the girls have brought inevitably go out, and the bolder boys grab the breasts of the girls. In retaliation, the girls strike the boys to ward them off, and may even knock them down.

Among the Western Apache of North America, there is a similar worry about improper attempts at seduction and the need for resistance on the part of girls, as told by Grenville Goodwin and Janice Thompson Goodwin.[3] A man knows not to touch a woman's breasts and also not her shoulders because of their proximity to the breasts, nor the legs or heels, which contact the girls private parts in the typical squatting posture. The girl is instructed by her parents not to run after boys, and not to let a man touch her body. This lecture from parents, is a typical one, and concerns themes of a girl's need to save herself for her future husband. For a man, touching the forbidden parts, if the woman is not his wife, is a recognized social offense for which he could be fined if the girl reports it. The exception to this rule occurs during acceptable love making, and with serious courting, at which times a suitor might be permitted to touch the girl's breasts and thighs. Thus the breasts are counted among the sexually responsive parts among the Apache as in other societies, and for the young Apache girl, as for the Italian American girl, and the Kapauku girl of Papua New Guinea, allowing the breasts to be fondled constitutes a possible danger.

Casual fondling of the breast is prohibited by the Cuna of Panama, for whom it is however allowed in bona fide premarital courtship, as with Sususappin and Turtle Woman's daughter. The Cuna are strict about discipline, and a girl who lets her breast be touched inappropriately commits a serious moral offense, according to Donald Stanley Marshall.[4] He cites an example at a military base where a group of Cuna people had gone to see a movie. A soldier was able to persuade a Cuna girl to let him touch her breast, and the next day she was sent by her community to an island for exile.

4

The breast in marriage and intercourse

EXCITATION OF THE BREASTS is a compelling force in the acts of married couples and lovers. A clay plaque of a couple embracing in a marriage bed from 2,000 BCE indicates the importance of the breast in marriage for the ancient people of Elam, which is present day Southwest Iran. See Figure 2.

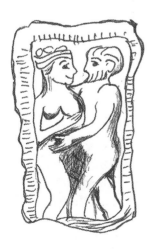

Figure 2
Embracing couple in marriage bed, clay plaque; c. 2000 BCE. Elam (Southwest Iran). Drawing by the author after a photo from the Louvre (Art Resource).

The erotic significance of the breast for both men and women among the Dogon people of Mali, West Africa is shown in several ways. In bed, a man expresses his sexual desire to a woman by touching her breasts, but the woman may make the first move. The words spoken between a husband and wife at night are called "speech of the breast". According to the metaphor, the breast in Dogon culture represents not only desire, but also communication. In Dogon society, young girls repeat songs about the breast, clapping their hands and singing that "speech of the night is speech of the breast in the night;" Genevieve Calame-Griaule, the ethnographer, notes that these songs are considered lewd, so there is no doubt of their sexual reference.[1] "Speech of the breast in the night" is also called "speech of desire". In Dogon culture, rape is referred to as "cutting the breast," which can be construed to mean that rape is sex without the involvement of the breasts, implying sex without a woman's consent.

Among the Aranda of central Australia, at the start of a new marriage, the wife returns to her mother every night for several nights. According to Geza Roheim, it is not until the wife overcomes her shyness with her husband and, after at first lying with her back to his, she turns and puts her leg over him enabling him to feel her breasts and her hair against him, that her husband knows that she desires him.[2] Turning toward the man and making the breasts available, as well as the genitals, is a recognized signal of an Aranda woman's sexual desire.

The breast, when offered by a woman to a man is an expression of her desire in Santal culture, as we have seen in various poems and folk songs. The breasts are also instrumental in obtaining climax. For example, in recounting the sex life of the Santals, Charulal Mukherjea tells us that not only do men handle a woman's breasts as a preliminary to sexual intercourse, but also during the sex act.[3] He notes that because the posture taken during coitus does not stimulate the breasts, they are squeezed with the man's hands. From Mukherjea's explanation, breast stimulation is desired and expected by the woman during coitus.

The following poem from the Santals indicates the relationship between a woman's desire, her breasts, and intercourse. Poem collected by William George Archer.[4]

> *Mongol, from the spring below the pond*
> *Pick the blossom for me.*
> *Like bel fruits are my breasts*
> *And you may take them.*
> *My mound is like a lamp*
> *And I will give it to you*
> *Utterly.* (98)

Not only may a man's hands perform the necessary breast play during coitus, as described above among the Santals, but a man's mouth on a woman's breasts is another way to bring her to climax. The following is related by Thomas Gladwin and Seymour B. Sarason concerning the people of Chuuk (Truk), an island of Micronesia, located north of Papua New Guinea.[5] The sex ritual is begun with the participants seated facing one another, and the two draw nearer to each other for intercourse. From this position, as they approach climax, he can kiss her and put his mouth on her body. Foreplay is not important for the Chuuk, but during coition, the breasts become engaged in the love act, according to Gladwin and Sarason, and the man's orgasm coincides with or follows that of the woman. This order, or ritual, of orgasm is meaningful, since, if the man's orgasm occurs first, the sex act ends prematurely, even if only temporarily. Notably the purpose of cultural sexuality is to enable woman's orgasm as well as man's. John Caughey indicates that, for the Chuuk, sexual intercourse is like a fight in which the partner who reaches climax last, is the winner.[6] He goes on to remark that when a woman does not reach orgasm, she chastises her lover for not being a man and advises him to "go like a baby and suck a breast."

The Mangaians, a Polynesian people from the Island of Mangaia in the central Pacific, were studied by Donald S. Marshall.[7] According to Marshall, in Mangaia, copulation is of great concern and

Mangaian women are known to always be able to achieve orgasm. Sexual training is given to young men by circumcision experts, and to young women by elderly women. They are instructed about such techniques as oral/genital sex, the kissing and sucking of breasts, and how to achieve mutual climax. The male is said to be taught to bring the woman to climax before allowing himself to achieve the goal. Although foreplay is brief, it includes lingual and manual caressing of breasts. Despite this intense and intimate sexuality or perhaps because of it, social contacts between male and female in the public sphere are not approved of. According to Marshall this includes public contact between husband and wife, brother and sister, old man and old woman, as well as sweethearts and lovers. However, for the young, secret rendezvous are easily agreed upon, and at age fourteen or fifteen there are groups of peers who discuss and encourage each other's sexual activities, but who only meet openly within the context of the community, at a picnic for instance.

Ralph Linton, in discussing the love affairs of the people of the Marquesan Islands in the central Pacific, said that these Polynesian people are extremely versed in erotic technique.[8] He provided a description of a typical erotic prelude in which the woman was dominant and the man acceded to her erotic desires. According to Linton the man's role was to arouse the woman by sucking her breasts and oral/genital contact. He further stated that the potency of a woman was reliant on these acts, without which she could not have an orgasm, a characteristic that he said was not uncommon in other primitive cultures. This assertion suggests that the use of the breasts to induce orgasm was a widespread phenomenon among preliterate societies.

The people of various cultures, from Africa, Australia, India and the Pacific Islands illustrate that in marital sex, women desire more than just a genital act. The work of Masters and Johnson showed that not only are the genitals involved in a woman's orgasm but also the breasts and the uterus,[9] and as discussed by Alice Rossi, there is an erotic tie between the breasts and the uterus.[10] Of course it is not necessary to understand the science to perform the act, but in the modern world it helps to know that breast stimulation during intercourse can physiologically induce orgasm.

In a study of contemporary educated men in the province of Inner Mongolia, China, it was found that only two out of twenty-one men in the city of Huhhot said they engaged in substantial foreplay that involved kissing and touching their spouse's lips and breasts. A report by William R. Jankowiak in 1993 described a man who felt responsible for his wife's inability to reach sexual orgasm, and asked his friends what he should do.[11] Their answer was that he should kiss his wife's breasts. Their suggestion did not result in a positive change for the couple because of complex reasons. But the fact that friends provided this information to the man is meaningful.

The above problem from present day China is a modern one manifesting itself in an urban setting. In an atmosphere of isolation from the extended family, which can be a locus of traditional knowledge and support, a woman may have no way to learn about cultural sexuality; it is not readily intuitive in a repressive society, and there is a sense of taboo about "unnatural" breast sex that is difficult to overcome in a male dominated technological milieu. Education concerning the erotic nature of the breasts would be beneficial to society, but the sexual use of the breasts still remains obscure to contemporary science. Hi-tech living has downgraded the status of the female breast from its once lofty position at the origin of *Homo sapiens*.

An account by Gerardo Reichel-Dolmatoff and Sydney Muirden describes the sex ritual of the Kogi, a tribe of the Sierra Nevada of Colombia, saying that, after a prelude of breast manipulation, coition is carried out facing one another, and the man is said to "eat" the woman.[12] This may have several meanings, but since the Kogi are talking about active coition, this suggests that the reference is to oral breast sex during intercourse. The Kogi have a myth, related by Reichel-Dolmatoff and Muirden, in which a jaguar pursues an adolescent girl and bites her on the breast.[13] She subsequently begins to growl like a jaguar, and, overcome by the ordeal, she dies. When her jaguar attacker is caught and killed, it is discovered that, instead of a paw, it has a human foot. The authors comment that fantasies of eating and being eaten are common in this type of myth, and refer to both hunger and thwarted sexuality.

Using a metaphor similar to that of the Kogi, when the Ashanti of Ghana talk of adultery or voluntary extramarital intercourse, they call it "eating" someone else's wife, as documented by Robert Sutherland Rattray.[14] This may be a reference to all types of sexual "eating," but easily included is a reference to the breast sex of traditional society. It is interesting to note that for the Hopi of Arizona the word "mama" is an expression meaning something to eat, including the breast, according to Wayne Dennis.[15]

From the Far East, two more instances of the role of the breast in marriage and intercourse are gathered. In their chapter on courtship, marriage, and sex in Okinawa, an island south of the Japanese mainland, we learn from Thomas Maretzki, Hatsumi Maretzki, and Beatrice B. Whiting that the breasts are considered to be sexual and for that reason men caress them.[16] In Korea, as told by Cornelius Osgood, on the evening of his marriage, the groom goes to the bride's house to hold her breasts.[17]

In the northern part of India, the Lepchas of Sikkim believe that no preliminary inducement is needed to start making love because sexual desire is thought to require no incentive, according to Geoffrey Gorer and J. H. Hutton.[18] But a Lepcha man will fondle a woman's breasts immediately before coition. Fondling of the breasts, if done in public, is thought to be an amusing but brazen act, since it is assumed to be directly related to sex. As among the Lepchas, there is extensive cultural understanding that touching the breasts is a sexual solicitation. The widespread nature of this conviction can be traced to the fact that the breasts are indeed erotic organs, and there are conventions and laws governing the touching of the breasts.

In discussing marriage and sex, one inevitably arrives at the topic of divorce. Among the Rungus Dusun of northern Borneo, Malaysia, at the time of marriage, men must pay a bride price, as reported by George N. Appell.[19] He states that the acknowledged purpose for the payment is to establish the husband's rights over the sexual services of his wife, and over her reproductive services. Sexual rights include the husband's rights to his wife's breasts. If the woman refuses to allow the man to exercise these rights, it is grounds for divorce. In a divorce case where a man has felt his wife's breasts, not all of the bride price is returned. If, in a marriage of short duration, the couple has had intercourse, only half of the bride price can be expected back, and if there is a child, none of the bride price is returnable. But in a marriage of longer duration, even though a woman is barren none of the bride price is returned. This is because, as explained by the Rungus people, the man has enjoyed a long period of sexual relations with her. Despite a man's right to touch his wife's breasts, to do so in public among the Rungus Dusun is considered improper. If he does not stop, the man's father-in-law can sue him for brassware as payment for improper contact of a woman's breasts.

Finally, a modern case study from the files of physician and sex psychologist Havelock Ellis, tells of a woman who frequently resorted to masturbation, perhaps because of marital dissatisfaction.[20] She reached orgasm by rubbing her genitals with one hand and her breasts with the other, ending by stimulating her breasts.

5

Denial of the sexual role of the breasts

IN TESTIMONY COLLECTED FROM several societies, the role of the breasts in producing sexual pleasure is minimized or denied. In the community of Bangkhuad, Thailand, Howard Keva Kaufman tells us that sexual intercourse between husband and wife – with the man always in the top position—involves fondling and kissing the breasts.[1] This happens except when a woman is lactating. However, Kaufman says that the women were almost unanimous in reporting that sex was mostly for the enjoyment of the man, not the woman. The word "mostly" points to the possibility that the women of Bangkhaud were perhaps being diffident about stating their own pleasure, which, at least was not nothing.

The following account by Suzette Heald concerning the Bagisu of Eastern Uganda is more definitive sounding, and we have less room for doubt, although perhaps some.[2] For the Bagisu, the physical relationship a woman has with her husband is clearly differentiated from the relationship she has with her children by ritual restrictions. Thus according to Heald, a man may never touch or suck his wife's breasts, as a child might do to its mother, under pain of ritual annulment and compensation. This outcome seems extreme, but perhaps it only pertains when the woman is breastfeeding her baby, as noted below.

Reminding us somewhat of the Bagisu of Africa, are the Garos of India. The Garos, are a tribal people who live north of Bangladesh in northeast India. There are several accounts of the sex life of the Garo, and these differ in detail. In one account by Tarunchandra Sinha, the author relates that although the men say they feel drawn to the bare breasts of the women, they claim that during sexual intimacies they do not press a woman's breasts because her breasts are meant for her child.[3] The author doubts this claim, saying that it is his belief that Garo men handle the breasts of women as much as do any other people. However, during lactation, especially in the early days or months after the birth of the child, the prohibition of sex is a known phenomenon in some African societies.

In another report concerning the Garo, authors M. C. Goswami and Dhirendra N. Majundar, found that as a preliminary to sexual intercourse the male may occasionally fondle the breasts of the female.[4] Among the villagers, unmarried sexually mature girls are not shy about keeping their breasts uncovered, and for a man to touch them is regarded as an erotic advance. Fondling or touching a married woman's breast by a man other than her husband is regarded as a transgression for which compensation must be paid. These stories indicate the nuances in acceptable sexual behavior that were kept track of regarding the breast.

For the San people, the hunter-gatherers of Botswana and also South Africa, among whom are the !Kung bushmen, breasts are associated with breast feeding, not sex, according to Lorna Marshall.[5] The !Kung are known to be exceedingly modest and do not expose their genitals, and the women do not expose their buttocks. According to Marshall, one reason for the modesty of the !Kung is that they are constantly in the presence of people with whom it is taboo to convey any expression of sexuality or eroticism. This has to do with the incest taboo and the fact that the !Kung band or village is small. However, Marshall reports that the breasts are kept bare for nursing.

Because they are constantly bare, breasts may present little stimulation to men of the San culture according to Ronald Singer.[6] However there is an aspect to a man's interest in his wife's breasts which has to do with sexual initiation. Singer notes that among the G/wi group of the San people, a girl marries between her seventh and ninth year to a man perhaps seven years her senior; since sexual intercourse does not begins till a few years later when the girl's breasts grow, her husband may become impatient if she is slow to develop. The correlation between the commencement of sexual intercourse and the development of a woman's breasts is the case here, and is found in many preliterate societies.

Marjorie Shostak reports that since the !Kung community is very small and usually only one girl matures at a time, she becomes a center of attention and her body is scrutinized by the men of the band, who comment on her bare breasts and joke about their desire to marry her.[7] Shostak tells of the thoughts of a young !Kung woman at the time of intercourse, and, meaningfully, her thoughts are of her breasts: of how they have become large, and of how she is "becoming a woman."

Among the G/wi group, the attitude toward intercourse is ambiguous; and George B. Silberbauer notes that it is considered improper for women to admit to enjoying sex.[8] However, one frequent complaint of G/wi women is that their husbands have little noticeable interest in initiating intercourse, which to Silberbauer indicates that the women enjoy it more than they are willing to admit.

Among the Manus people of New Guinea, the ultimate form of disrespect is copulation, as related by Margaret Mead.[9] This would seem to relegate marriage for the Manus to a very unpleasant affair. The relationship between husband and wife is usually tense and reserved, and women angrily refute the idea that their husbands touch their breasts, according to Mead.[10] She does say however that all her remarks on sex must be qualified because the Manus are such a puritanical people that it is difficult to trust any information they give about intimate sex.[11]

Oddly, while it is forbidden to play with a wife's breasts in marriage, the wedding trip to the husband's house is called "the journey of the breasts," and immediately after the marriage, as described by Mead, there is an unusual amount of commentary in the groom's village on the breasts of his new bride.[12] Mead characterizes the relationship between husband and wife as unaffectionate, perhaps as might be expected considering the strange attitude of the Manus to coitus and the breast.

However, in contrast to the reserved relationship between husband and wife, there is a special relationship in the culture of Manus between some cousins, called a joking relationship, which is described by Reo Fortune.[13] Curiously this relationship involves playing with a woman's breasts – a kind of playful disrespect according to Fortune between a man and his father's sister's daughter.

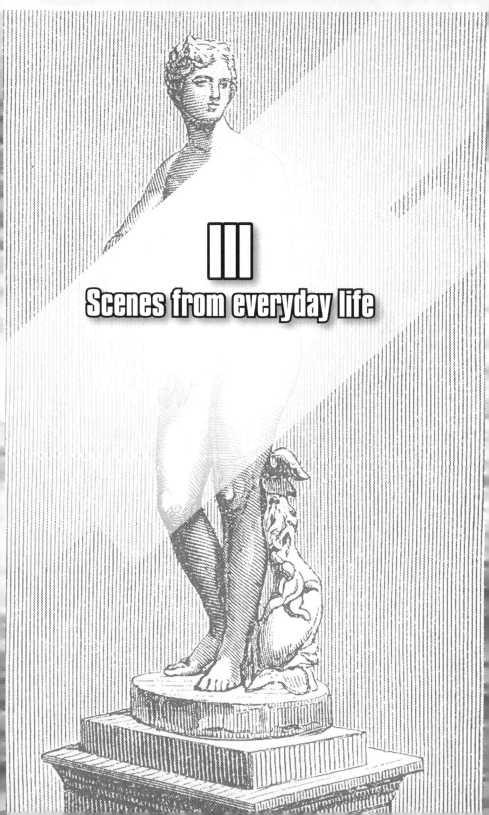

III
Scenes from everyday life

1

Humor, sex, and the breast

SEX AMUSES PEOPLE, AND though we hardly need to be convinced of this, examples from a few ethnic groups provide glimpses into what was entertaining in simpler times. One such group are the Iban a branch of the Dyak people of Borneo. In this culture it was perfectly acceptable while joking with young women of the community in a playful setting, for young men to hold them around the waist and try to touch their breasts, as reported by Hugh Brooke Low and H. Ling Roth.[1] In a modern setting this would strike us as harassment, but sexual teasing between the sexes is portrayed as acceptable among the Iban, at least in 1892.

Sex is always funny to the Lepchas of the Himalayan state of Sikkim, India, according to Geoffrey Gorer and J. H. Hutton.[2] They describe a party where there is considerable drinking and where obscene remarks occasion a great deal of laughter. Some practical jokes are perpetrated, and a certain amount of rough sexual play occurs. Young men make grabbing gestures at other young men's genitals, and once in a while a young woman will do so as well. Bolder young men try to fondle the breasts of the young married women, but are repulsed with extreme actions such as a slap in the face, which the men accept as part of the game.

There is a story of drinking and playing at a Lepcha religious festival as told by John Morris.[3] At the festivities, a boy of about sixteen tried to feel the breasts of a villager's wife, to the amusement of onlookers and the woman herself. After she freed herself from his attempted embrace, she bared her breast, squeezed milk from it and ran after the boy trying to rub the milk in his face.

The drum dance of the Copper Inuit of the central Canadian Arctic is an occasion for joking and horsing around. As described by Duncan Pryde, people who gather for an evening of dancing, get in the mood by first having some fun.[4] At one particular event described by Pryde, the preliminaries consisted of three men, each with a baby's bottle filled with milk and capped with a nipple, competing to see who could empty his bottle first. This produced much laughter and commentary by the women. According to Pryde, a woman named Irvana shouted to the others to look at one of the contestants. She said that she wouldn't mind "having him at her breast." Here is an apparent reference to woman's sexuality of the breast, although, in this case, with a humorous allusion. Another woman joined in the fun, asking what kind of husbands these men would make – that they were just big babies. She wondered what such men could do for a woman – how such big babies could make children.

Among the Serbs there is a story with elements similar to the Copper Inuit story, but with a slightly different twist. As related by Andrei Simic, an old grandfather remembers when he was a child hearing his aunts laughing and joking about their husbands.[5] They repeated a common Serb aphorism, used by women, that says that as long as he lives, a man is like a child, and that to keep him contented, you must keep him at your breast.

Among the Navaho, there are always humorists who want to make people laugh according to Willard W. Hill.[6] Hill tells the story of a man, his wife, and two other people who took a one-day trip to Zuni, returning the next day. The woman left her young nursing child at home, and on the way back her breasts began to hurt. This forced the party to stop. To relieve her, her husband began to suckle her breasts. He then tried to turn the act into a humorous imitation of sex for the benefit of the others in the group, but at this juncture, the wife pushed her husband away. The wife seems to have been complicit in the joke up to a point, which brings up the observation that in communities based on kinship or where the extended family is strong, there is an openness about human sexuality that in a more complex society is demeaning to women.

2

The breasts and joking among relatives

AT THE RISK OF appearing to present a mere catalogue of sexual behaviors, the following descriptions of mostly tribal customs are provided to reduce the dearth of information about cultural sexuality and its reliance on the breast. It clarifies our analysis of our own sexual practices if we compare them with those of people from other times and locales, even those which might be considered abusive today.

Among the Manus people of New Guinea, Margaret Mead reports that between a man and his female cross cousin, that is, his father's sister's daughter, public jesting is allowed, characterized by jocular talk by the man and his right to touch the woman's body, including her breasts in a playful way.[1] According to Mead, the joking is permitted only in public, and over-indulgence is construed as an offense. One or both of the cousins is usually married, and the playing is definitely sexual. But sexual intercourse between them is taboo, and is reserved only for husband and wife. The report does not reveal whether the woman can take liberties with the man's body.

Where life span is short and the death of a spouse a concern, permitting sexual familiarities of the breast is a way to prepare for a possible new marriage. The sororate is a marriage system in which a widower is expected to marry a sister of his deceased wife, according to Dennis O'Neil.[2] He says that in places where polygyny, or marriage to more than one woman is popular, and where it is possible for a man's wives to be sisters, a married woman may encourage some sexual behavior between her husband and her sister because she would prefer that her sister rather than another woman marry her husband if she dies. Maintenance of an existing bond between two families is one rationale, as well as to insure the well being of children in case of parental death. A related marriage system is the levirate, in which a widow can or should marry her deceased husband's brother. The practice has been recorded in many societies across the world – in Africa, the Middle-East, Central Asia, and North America – with some degree of sexual access allowed in certain cultures in anticipation of a presumed marriage.

The Lozi people of Zambia, Africa, practice a marriage system of polygyny in which co-wives have relatively equal status, each living in a separate dwelling. Some of the kinship relations and joking practices of the Lozi are explained by Max Gluckman, including joking with children.[3] An uncle on the mother' side, that is, a mother's brother, may refer to his young niece as his wife, and to his nephew as co-husband. Also a father's sister, may call her niece her co-wife, and her nephew her husband. Because the relationships are friendly and jocular, the young people can easily consult these elders on sexual matters. This terminology ceases when the children grow up, except in the case of uncle and nephew, at which time the nephew can sleep in his uncle's hut, touch the breasts of his uncle's wife, and, if his uncle dies, marry his wife if she is willing. Teasing between grandparents and grandchildren of the opposite sex also occurs among the Zambian Lozi, and they can address each other as co-husband and co-wife.

Among the Saramaka of Suriname, South America, who are of African descent, the grandparents and others of their generation can joke with the grandchildren's generation about sex. The genitals and breast area of little girls can be jokingly touched by these men, and a little boy's penis can be tugged at by the women, as elucidated by Sally Price.[4]

The Santal tribal group of India maintain joking relationships between a man and his wife's younger sisters. They can call each other names, talk openly, and joke, as reported by W. J. Culshaw.[5] Similar interactions, as well as intimacies of the breast, take place between a woman and her husband's younger brothers. On the other hand a woman must behave with utmost deportment in front of her husband's older brother. These various levels of socializing are well understood by all tribal members.

Continuing with the Santals, the relationship of grandparents to grandchildren is a joking one according to Culshaw, and reflects deep intimacy and love. He says the situation arises because the children are often left in the care of their grandparents while parents go to work. Marine Carrin-Bouez and John Beierle further explain this relationship of the Santals, saying that the grandparents of both sexes are responsible for the cultural education of their grandchildren, and grandmothers can go so far as to sexually initiate grandsons.[6] On the other hand, according to Culshaw, children must behave with deference toward those of their parents' generation, addressing them with relationship terms rather than names.

Among the Tarahumara, a native American people of the Sierra Madre in Mexico, rough play may take place between kin, as reported by John G. Kennedy.[7] This is a variation of a joking relationship and sometimes may be used as a chance to bully a kins-person under the pretext of an accepted interaction. Kennedy describes the scene of a drunken teenager holding a close kinswoman around the breasts and pushing her to the ground. Between men, wrestling is one way to conduct this type of playing, sometimes leading to insults and fights and sexual comments. A joking relationship with sexual overtones can also take place between grandparents and grandchildren of the Tarahumara, and rough playing may be seen especially between a grandmother and her granddaughter.

In his study of Serbian alternative social structures and ritual relations in the Balkans of Europe, Eugene A. Hammel notes that sexual access is implied regarding relations between a man and his brother's wife, particularly a bride.[8] After the marriage, the groom's brother is often said to take sexual liberties with the bride, as related by Hammel in the case of a husband's brother who was teased about fondling his sister-in-law's breasts. Such a relationship may be a joking one, but Hammel says that more complete sexual contact may take place between men and their brother's wives. Such intimate relationships are sometimes occasioned by migrant labor jobs that take men away for long periods of time, and may go beyond the joking relationship. Also there may be sexual relations between a father and his son's wife. This happens when, to exempt the son from certain levies, the son is married at a young age to an older woman. These father/daughter-in-law relationships are more often regarded as sinful, than brother/sister-in-law relationships.

3

Kinship and breast taboos

FROM ETHNOGRAPHIC ACCOUNTS WE learn that sex taboos are associated with exogamy, a practice which specifies that marriage is forbidden with certain close relatives. Roy Franklin Barton writes about the Ifugao people of the Philippines, who practice exogamy and observe relevant taboos.[1] For instance in the presence of male and female kin with whom marriage is forbidden, it is taboo to refer unnecessarily to matters connected with sex or to look fixedly at a woman's breasts or hips.

For the Ganda of Uganda, Africa, as described by John Roscoe, a man's mother-in-law is taboo to him.[2] A mother-in-law must cover her face when passing her son-in-law, and he, at the same time, must take a detour to give her the path. If he sees her breasts he must give her a present of cloth to conceal them, or else some illness might strike him. Roscoe depicts similar avoidance behavior for the Banyoro, a neighboring tribe of the Ganda.[3] For the Banyoro, any communication a man has with his mother-in-law has to be from a distance, and he must look the other way if she happens to pass.

Among the Bagisu, another tribe of Uganda, prohibitive behavior is motivated by the fear of sexual contact, according to Suzette Heald, and concentrates on not touching certain individuals or seeing them naked.[4] This is the case for mother-in-law/son-in-law relationships of the Bagisu. The men say that they respect and honor their mother-in-laws, and are afraid they might find them beautiful.

The Zulu of South Africa require that a new bride must observe avoidance rules with respect to her father-in-law, as reported by Otto Friedrich Raum.[5] She must not be where her father-in-law is, and if she meets him by chance she must step aside or go into a hut. She must also hide her face and avoid looking at him. The cloth over her shoulders is made to cover her breasts because she must not have her breasts exposed in his presence. These rules are observed until the bride is ritually released from them.

Thomas Gladwin and Seymour B. Sarason explain that, as youngsters, the Chuuk of the western Pacific become aware that kinship terms for a group of relatives provide cues for the proper behavior toward them.[6] Many of these terms are the same as those used for the immediate family. Thus all the men in one's father's generation are termed father, and the all women in one's mother's generation are termed mother. Sexual intercourse and even mention of sexual subjects is prohibited between a man and anyone he calls mother. For a woman the same prohibition applies with anyone she calls father, with the added rule that she must never allow him to see her exposed breasts. For the group of children who are termed brother and sister strict provisions begin to be observed with the onset of sexual maturity. A brother should not be seen in the company of, or sleep in the same house with a sister. He should not see the exposed breasts of a sister, nor allow any sexual references to enter into a conversation with her. The sister also has an obligation to prevent the forbidden behavior.

Like the Chuuk of Oceania, the Navaho of North America maintain strong taboos against physical contact between mature sisters and brothers. Dorothea Cross Leighton and Clyde Kluckhohn investigated the relationship between opposite sex siblings among the Navaho.[7] They note the community gossip about incest, and that in the isolated circumstances in which most Navaho children grow up, there is a budding sexual attraction between sister and brother which must be curtailed. They feel that the popular mating arrangement among the Navaho, in which a brother and sister from one family marry a sister and brother from another, is an unconscious substitution for incestuous wishes. Training in avoidance of physical contact begins early and is extreme. Boys are told if they see up their sister's skirt they will go blind and they are told not to touch their sisters. After marriage, a brother must not see his sister's breasts, so that if she is nursing her child in the same hogan, she must keep covered.

We saw in the previous section that sex games involving the breast are permitted between certain in-laws among the Santals for whom sex with relatives is regulated under the law. There also exist taboos regarding the breast. For instance, if a woman is unmarried she must keep her breasts covered in the presence of a brother-in-law, nor can she mount a ladder or climb a tree in his presence according to William George Archer.[8]

A folksong of the Santals collected by Charulal Mukherjea also attests to the breast prohibition.[9] In it, a young man asks his sister-in-law to place his hand on her breast. He pleads with her to "raise" his hand to her breast. She replies that she could do this, but wonders what if "by chance my bracelets and anklets should jangle," and says, what "if by chance your brother catches us."

When the Santals engage in hunting wild game, some rules of sexual conduct are relaxed according to Archer in his book, *The Hill of Flutes*.[10] Archer comments that it would be amazing if girls and boys were never attracted by forbidden relatives. He goes on to say that it is natural that sometimes family fondness is replaced with a feeling that is stronger between an aunt younger than her nephew, or between an uncle and his niece. He discusses the difficulties brought about by the sexual repression demanded under ordinary circumstances. The hunt provides time when at least joking about sex can take place and wild stories can be told. This relaxed behavior alleviates forbidden desires according to Archer. And it would seem that despite prohibitions, forbidden sexual liaisons occur.

Mukherjea provides us with a verse for this situation in *The Santals.*[11] Here the young man asks his sister-in-law how coition is accomplished. She tells him that it is done by "sitting on the ground" and she describes thighs placed on thighs or against each other. Then she advises him to continue by "pressing" the woman's breasts and "gently moving" his body.

4

Sex education from infancy to puberty and beyond

IN VARIOUS FAR FLUNG cultures, parents' concern with the sexual education of their children extends from the child's infancy to the time of puberty and sexual initiation. During childhood children learn much by observation and interaction, while at initiation ceremonies adults of the community perform rituals and instruct children in sexual matters. There are even instances where older relatives perform the coital initiation of children.

We learned from Sally Price, in the context of joking among kin, that the Saramaka or Maroons who live along the Suriname River in the northern Amazon forest, have a tradition of grandparents touching children's genitals and the undeveloped breasts of little girls.[1] Adults are amused when three or four year olds play at sexual intercourse. This behavior, in a loving family milieu, is meant to be educational – teaching children about their sexuality. The Maroons successfully escaped from slavery as early as the 1500's, bringing with them the culture and ways of Africa.

The same methods of sex education are practiced by the Copper Inuit of far northern Canada, where children fondle and play with one another, and parents urge them on, according to Raymond DeCoccola.[2] He notes that Eskimo children observe their parents in all aspects of lovemaking, and in imitation of their parents, they can be heard during their childhood sex games exclaiming how wonderful it is.

Other examples of touching and teasing are known. For instance, Jean E. Jackson says that among the Tukano Indians of Colombia, women will manipulate the genitals of children.[3] Similar acts include a mother's fondling of her baby's penis while he is breast-feeding, as seen among the Navaho by Clyde Kluckhohn.[4] This last activity must make nursing an erotic experience for the child, suggesting one reason why men are enamored of the female breast.

As can be seen from the above, children, in some situations are thought of as little lovers. The opposite also happens. The equating of lovers with little babies occurs in Navaho and Eskimo humor, as has been described, and also among the Iban of North Borneo. For the Iban this can be seen in the context of an incantation that is sometimes used by a woman to entice a man to love her. If she desires a man, but he does not love her, she makes an offering to several fairy goddesses, who provide her with a love potion. In her prayer she asks that it might affect the man of her dreams, causing him to behave like an infant who desires her breast. This account is from William Howell.[5]

Among the Aranda of central Australia, the transition from childhood to adulthood is accomplished by an initiation ceremony for both girls and boys. The female breasts have a role in these proceedings. Herbert Basedow describes the ritual for a girl, which takes place when she first shows signs of adolescence.[6] It is a simple ceremony compared to the one for a boy. The husband to whom the girl has been assigned, along with other tribal men who lawfully will enjoy some sexual privileges with her, gently bring her a short distance from the camp. Her future husband then anoints each of her breasts with grease and with a circle of red ochre. Meanwhile, the others, who act as enchanters, sing to summon up the girl's womanly qualities and to coax her breasts to grow. From time to time the men place their lips on her nipples as if trying to draw them out. These actions, in addition to bidding the breasts to grow, embody a reference to future sexuality of the breast.

An Aranda boy's initiation rites, according to George Peter Murdock are complicated and can be painful and dangerous.[7] They are designed to test his manhood and his willingness to obey elders and observe tribal customs. The rituals, which involve the mother's breasts, are described by Geza Roheim.[8] The mothers take the sons by the hand and lead them to fires built by the fathers on which are piled green bushes. The initiates must stand on the bushes, which emit a heavy smoke. In one tribe of the Aranda, after the trial by fire and smoke, among other complex proceedings, the mothers go up and rub their nipples on their sons' mouths. In another tribe, when the novices return from the fire, they eat a seed preparation mixed with mother's milk. In still another tradition, the mothers offer their breasts, which the novices pretend to suck. In these ceremonies, the female breast plays a significant part, whether denoting good-byes or intimations of future sexuality with wives.

A custom among the Santals of India is reminiscent of the Aranda initiation ceremony. On saying good-bye to his mother on the day he departs for his bride's village and his wedding ceremonies, the son pretends to suckle her breasts, according to William George Archer.[9] In payment the mother receives a rupee from him which is deemed to be the price of her breasts. In this way is ended his intimate association with his mother, as he prepares to form a new intimate relationship with his wife.

Another story of approaching manhood and mother's breasts comes from the Lepchas of the Himalayas and is told by John Morris.[10] The age at which children are weaned there, can be surprisingly late. Some boys may be nursed until just before puberty. In this story, a boy who is old enough to hike some distance from his mother to see the natural sights of the area, returns to her and begins to suckle her breasts. She addresses him, asking what he saw. Upon learning that he saw some beautiful birds she refers to his impending adolescent sexuality and tells him that he must catch the birds to show that he is a man.

5

Breasts and the law

FONDLING THE BREASTS IS a standard way for a man to solicit sex, and when the act is done against the wishes of a woman, she is considered a victim. In present day United States, the 2003 U.S. Code of Law, Title 42 regarding Public Health and Welfare, in Chapter 147 concerning Prison Rape Elimination, the term "sexual fondling" is defined to mean touching the private parts of another person including the breasts and the genitalia, and adjacent areas, for the purpose of sexual gratification. It legally addresses prison rape, either prisoner on prisoner, or by a prison employee, a situation in which women prisoners are especially vulnerable.

Several instances of the illegality of fondling the breasts, as well as the fines that may be levied, can be found in the anthropological record. In Kapauku society of New Guinea, as described by Leopold Pospisil, a boy of about seventeen years of age saw a girl drawing water from the river.[1] He chased her and held her breasts, trying to get her to acquiesce to sexual intercourse. When the girl screamed and hit him, he let her go out of fear. The case was brought before the authorities, and the girl's father asked for compensation. Pospisil identified the act of holding the woman's breasts as an attempted seduction.

According to Robin Fox, most systems of family law exist to protect marriage from the emotional whims of individuals.[2] Depending on the culture, indemnity can be demanded, that is, compensation or reimbursement for acts that are considered sexual transgressions. In some societies the fine associated with public fondling of breasts applies only if the woman is the wife of another man. In Borneo among the Iban people, as pointed out by Hugh Brooke Low and H. Ling Roth, when men are joking and laughing with girls, it is no offense for the men to squeeze the girls' breasts, whereas it is an offense involving a fine to do this to a married woman.[3]

The law of the Rungus Dusun in north Borneo says that if a man takes hold of a woman's breasts a charge may be brought against the man. According to Laura Appell, the offense requires the offender to pay the victim a piece of brassware.[4] A person can also be sued for secretly looking at someone's genitals or watching sexual intercourse. In one case related by Appell, a man fondled a woman's breasts in the longhouse, but because the woman too had committed a sexual offense by secretly peeping at him earlier, the two offenses cancelled each other out. In Rungus society, it is clear that if a woman's breasts are touched in marriage, she has rendered a sexual service to her husband, and even if the marriage is otherwise unconsummated and he divorces her, he must pay compensation.

The following story is from the Santal of India. At a festival a boy caught the breasts of a girl, and when he did so she turned on him and called him a "bidhua" or bastard as described by William G. Archer.[5] As the story goes, the village council was called and at the meeting they decided that although the boy made an advance on her, it didn't warrant the girl's use of the insulting term. She, rather than the boy, was fined a rupee and four annas.

Among the Alorese, as mentioned earlier, pulling the breasts is a euphemism for sexual intercourse. In the following account from Cora DuBois, Abram Kardiner, and Emil Oberholzer, during litigation involving several families, a woman denied having intercourse with the husband of another, but when she admitted that he pulled her breasts, this was considered an admission of intercourse.[6] The man was called in and a judgment was made against him of five rupiah moko, which he paid.

Sexual offenses were listed by Robert Sutherland Rattray for the Ashanti tribe of Ghana, Africa.[7] Most serious was adultery, which was described idiomatically as "eating" someone else's wife. As we saw, this is the same expression used for the act by the Kogi tribe of the Sierra Nevada. Among other possibilities, this idiom can be construed as a reference to oral stimulation of the breasts. Of course, it could refer to both oral/genital and breast sex. Pulling at a woman's breasts was another sexual offense for the Ashanti, as well as several other activities associated with trying to seduce a woman.

In Mongolia the treatment of women as of the 1930s, differed within and outside of the home according to Valentin A. Riasanovsky.[8] Within the family, the patriarchal mode of life meant that women were subordinate to men, and they were sometimes dealt with harshly at the discretion of the male head of household. This might even mean the killing of a rejected wife, according to Riasanovsky. However, outside the family, humane principles were in evidence. For instance men were punished for licentious sexual behavior with women and girls. A case in point is the levying of a fine and some other punishments inflicted for kissing a girl over ten years of age, or touching her breasts.

6

The breast at dances and ceremonies

WOMEN'S BREASTS RECEIVE SPECIAL attention during dance performances and at certain ritual ceremonies and celebratory occasions where there is a sexual aspect. For some celebrations women paint their breasts to make them beautiful and enticing. For instance, Tukano women of South America paint red circles on their breasts for dancing, according to Alcionilio da Silva and Ivana Lillios;[1] and Aranda women of Australia paint stripes from their shoulders to their knees for the wuljankura dance according to Geza Roheim, which includes the breasts.[2] Silva notes the attraction that Tukano men have for women's breasts. This trait is no doubt shared by men the world over, given sexual associations and the way that women unabashedly display them at certain times.

Breasts entertain, as in the so-called entertainment dances or shoulder dances of the Amhara of Ethiopia. These are performed by professionals at crowded venues, as described by Simon D. Messing, and the crowd may join in the dance.[3] Here, the shoulders are moved in a circular and back and forth movement to the beat of a drum; each movement is accompanied by a hissing sound of air drawn though the teeth. If a woman is performing, she may introduce an additional element into the motion, thrusting her breasts forward, and bouncing a dangling cross from breast to breast.

A Santal dance of India described by W. G. Archer, has characteristics similar to the Amharic performance.[4] Girls and young women dance to the beat of drums, and their motions progress from slow undulation in the first round to wild and undisciplined movement in the final round. The drummers meanwhile beat ever faster and begin to toss their drums about; they accompany this with snake-like hissing, and jerking head movements. At the height of the dance, the girls leap up and down with erratic motions and let their breasts bounce. They finally collapse into laughter and talking.

Individuals are sometimes identified as flirts because of their behavior. Just so, a particular young woman of the Mbuti always showed off her breasts at dances, gathering admiring looks from the bachelors, as described by Colin Turnbull.[5] Turnbull wrote an account of the Mbuti hunter-gatherers, the pygmies of the Congo rainforest, and in his story of the flirtatious young woman, he predicts that her initiation festival, the elima, will be a lively event, when she will choose one of the bachelors to spend the night with her.

Dancing is part of a ritual ceremony of the Cubeo Indians, a branch of the Tukano culture of South America. The event lasts several days, and sexual license is the outcome. The theme of the dramatization is the changing sexual interplay of men and women throughout life, and it starts with a mourning ceremony as described by Irving Goldman.[6] From its solemn beginnings, abandon sets in. During the dancing on the second day, there is laughter, playing, and throwing of mash. Then masked male dancers fall upon the participating women. The men do not touch the women with their hands, but ritually jostle them, as if accidentally. However, young boys at the dance, become aroused, and in the confusion, they fall among the women to clutch at their breasts.

Another ritual of the Tukano in which the breast is featured, is the yurupari fertility ceremony, as described by Gerardo Reichel-Dolmatoff.[7] It is a celebration at which there is an interchange of marriageable women between two groups of the Tukano culture, and is marked by the playing of flutes and trumpets by the men. After the available women and girls file into the longhouse, they are followed by the men carrying meat, fruit and nettles. With shoving and joking the men stage a sham battle with the women, touching the women on the breasts and on the back with meat and fruit or with the nettles. The women laugh and pretend to flee, while allowing themselves to be touched by the men. After a while the food is eaten, and there is drinking and dancing. The first part of the ritual is meant to be threatening, representing the separation of the sexes, and the second part is joyful, representing their union.

The Western Apaches of North America are extremely modest according to Grenville Goodwin and Janice T. Goodwin.[8] The authors tell of the following incident that depicts the typical modesty of the young women. Adolescent girls, who had been surprised by an enemy while swimming, had to escape without their clothes. On the way back to camp, they made skirts of willow branches, and they also held willow branches in front of them to cover their breasts.

For the Western Apache, exposed breasts indicate sexual abandon. At victory celebrations for returning warriors, unmarried women, such as widows and divorcees, dance clothed only with a small apron and a thin piece of cloth around their breasts according to Grenville Goodwin and Keith Basso.[9] Married women and girls would not have exposed their breasts and bodies in this way. The warriors are honored by the dancing, during which the women thank them for killing an enemy. The women do not dance for nothing and they request gifts such as a blanket or cloth from the victory spoils. Such celebrations are followed by a night of sexual abandon.

In the Aranda culture of Australia, as described by Geza Roheim, at special festivals there is a woman's dance called the waljankura, carried out to incite female desire for men other than their husbands.[10] The dance ends with an exchange of spouses. Early in the festivities, a woman gives her husband the name of the person with whom she would like to have intercourse, and he arranges the exchange. Women and girls rub their bodies with grease and paint themselves in preparation for the dance and love-making. The term waljankura refers to a greased person. According to Roheim, the women and girls dance until their legs tremble with excitement. At the performance, the girls sing very loudly and their breasts are also said to "sing very loudly," a concept reminiscent of the African Dogon people's "speech of the breast in the night", a metaphor for desire.

Apropos the characterization of the breasts as capable of speech and song, the Navajo have a myth about Changing Woman and her creation of the first man and the first woman. Maureen Trudelle Schwartz recounts the story of how the man's penis is made of turquoise and the woman's vagina has a red shell clitoris.[11] When Changing Woman places the organs side by side and commands them to shout, the penis shouts, but not the vagina. Changing Woman commands them to have intercourse and to try shouting again. When they try again, the penis is weak, but the vagina has a very good shouting voice.

For Zulu girls, exposed breasts are a sign of moral decency according to Eileen Jensen Krige.[12] A girl is proud of her breasts and, in contrast to the Navajo, she is given many opportunities to display them. After having reached maturity, when attending dances for the first time, girls may appear almost naked except for a few beads or leaves. If a girl covers her breasts at a dance, it is a sign of a loose sexual life. For a virgin, her nakedness is a sign of her purity, while for a married woman, it is a sign of debasement.

Women of the San, known on most occasions for their modesty, dance naked at the time of a girl's first menstruation ceremony as described by Jiro Tanaka.[13] The only covering is a small apron over the pubic area. However no men are in attendance – they are not permitted. The women of the camp surround the hut in which the girl is isolated and they shed their clothes and dance what is known as the eland dance. According to Tanaka, they proudly exhibit their prominent buttocks, and swing and bounce their breasts in celebration.

7

Some attributes of the breast

THE ORIGINAL FUNCTION OF the female breast is to provide nutrition for the young of the mammalian species. The milky mammary gland is the definitive organ of the mammal, and just as the young are kept nearby and protected, so too, the mammary glands lie close to and under the trunk of the female quadruped body. In the case of the quadrupedal chimpanzee, the breasts are not curvaceous with fatty tissue, as in the human female, and even when lactating the chimp's breasts are only slightly enlarged, imparting a flat-chested appearance. Theories abound as to why women's milk glands are covered with a layer of fat just under the skin, making the breasts into soft rounded hemispheres. Citing the Northern Anthropological Association, Elaine Morgan in her book *The Descent of Woman*, names three advantages of the fatty insulating layer of the breast: it provides a cushion above the more fragile sub-tissue, it helps to keep the milk warm, and it serves to store a reserve of calories.[1] With the advent of bipedalism the arms began to be used to carry sticks and other objects used for tools and weapons, and cold weather was possible even in the warm climate where humans evolved. Our upright human posture and related activity, in a major way, exposes the milk glands to injury and also to the weather.

Fat insulation around the breasts, while influencing general upper body temperature, also helps to regulate the temperature of breast milk. A nursing infant may be at the breast for varying lengths of time, from months to several years, determined more or less by the prevailing culture. As the infant suckles, milk forms in the milk glands, but often the so called milk let-down reflex allows milk to fill the breasts more quickly. A delay in nursing can leave the breasts very full, and the milk can be affected by the ambient temperature. Living in a cold climate or where the weather is variable can create a problem for a nursing mother.

Even in moderate climates, nights can be cold, and high on mountain sides in moderate and even hot climates, there may be snow and freezing weather, as in Africa and elsewhere. Melvin Konner mentions the freezing temperatures during winter in the bush in connection with the hazards that a lost San child of Botswana would endure.[2] These same hazards threaten a nursing mother.

In such circumstances, and in year round cold environments, there is a danger of breast-milk freezing. In quadrupeds, the location of the breasts under the body affords some shielding from the weather by the four legs. But even for a dog in the sub-zero cold of the polar north, breast milk will freeze. Raymond DeCoccola tells the story of the Eskimo woman, Oviluk, who had forgotten to attach the apron of caribou skin, used as a blanket, over her nursing dog's belly.[3] The dog was almost entirely lacking in hair around the nipples, and the milk in the breasts had frozen solid. Oviluk, whose own breasts were full because her four year old daughter had not been weaned, declared that she had enough milk for her daughter and for the two newborn pups, and she nursed one pup and then the other under her parka. Presumably the warm igloo in which she resided, as well as her parka, provided protection to her own breast milk.

There is another culture in which we encounter the freezing of the breasts, perhaps more in the sense of a frozen capability to produce milk. The idea that repeatedly exposing the breasts to cold weather will prevent the breasts from making milk is found among the Hopi according to Mischa Titiev.[4] He relates the story of a childless woman, Ida, of the Hopi of Arizona, who was told that even if she did have a child, she would not be able to suckle it because, on various occasions in Flagstaff where she worked, she had gone outdoors with only very light clothing. A perusal of the weather conditions in Flagstaff reveal that, despite predominantly mild weather, temperatures often fall steeply after sunset, and winter nights can be extremely cold.

In the relatively hairless human condition there is no body hair to which the young can cling, if need be. The young of chimps, on the other hand, can cling to the mother's fur when she is on the move. A function of the breasts therefore, which occurs among the Aranda of Australia according to Herbert Basedow, is to provide handles for the baby to hold on to when the mother is occupied.[5] He describes a woman making her way through the environment in search of food, with her child in her arms securing itself by holding on to one or both of her breasts. He notes that this contributes to the sagging appearance of the breasts of older women.

The female breasts are associated with sexuality in cultures throughout the world. Under the influence of female hormonal control, the milk glands of the breast begin to mature early in puberty, and at the same time the associated fat deposits give the breasts their characteristic shape. The layer of fat underlying much of our bodily surface is discussed by Ronald Singer, who writes about the biology of the San people.[6] He notes that fat tends to accumulate in certain parts of the body such as the hips, abdomen, inner thighs, and arms in both sexes, and in the breasts of women. Particularly in the breasts, the fat layer assumes a shape in women that is sexually stimulating.

Something as basic as gravity, acting on mammary fat deposits, contributes to the appealing hemispherical and somewhat dropped shape of the breasts in young women, and to a more pendulous shape later on. According to the theory of sexual selection as described by Geoffrey Miller, the preference of men for shapely female breasts has influenced the mammary contours of women.[7] In this case, men more often choose as mates the women who have a preferred breast shape.

8

Beliefs about maturation of the breasts

THE BREASTS START TO develop in association with puberty and with general sexual maturation. However, in some cultures it is thought that the maturation of the breasts must be induced by sexual activity. In other words, a girl's entry into womanhood is due to the involvement of men. In these cases, as explained by several anthropologists, men appear to arrogate to themselves the credit for womanhood.

The Lepchas of the Himalayas do not recognize or have a word for puberty, as reported by Geoffrey Gorer and J. H. Hutton.[1] Instead they believe that the swelling of the breasts and the beginning of the menses are the result of copulation, and that therefore girls must indulge in sexual intercourse in order to mature. Some women report having had sex at ten or eleven years old, and occasionally a man will force a girl of this age to have sex. There is no stigma attached to this activity, because it is felt that girls are dependent on the intervention of men to make them mature. If a virgin starts to exhibit signs of puberty, a supernatural being is said to have visited her. Gorer and Hutton comment that this supposed intercession by men in women's

Valerie Robinson

maturation, or this cultural explanation for a physiological process, may be due to an extreme envy that men feel for women's life giving processes. They note that this may be so in some tribes of New Guinea and Australia as well as in the Himalayas.

In the Pacific island culture of Chuuk, puberty is culturally defined for girls by the appearance of their first menses, which usually occurs later than the first signs of breast development, as recounted by Gladwin and Sarason.[2] These authors make the observation that intercourse is supposedly prohibited until puberty, but since it is widely believed by the Chuuk that intercourse aids in the growth of a girl's breasts and the onset of her menstruation, the honoring of the prohibition appears rather questionable. According to Ward Hunt Goodenough, Chuuk girls start to have intercourse at about age fourteen when their breasts are somewhat developed.[3] Marc J. Swartz cites a Chuuk guide who informed him that when a man notices that a girl is becoming a woman, with breasts that are beginning to develop, it incites him to desire intercourse with her, whether or not he believes that female development is furthered by copulation.[4] According to Gladwin and Sarason, boys and girls both have a fair amount of sexual experience by the time they are sixteen, and Goodenough states that there is no shame felt about adolescent sex before marriage.

Marriage among the Bororo Indians of the Amazon Basin of Brazil is typically between a man and a girl as reported by Zarko David Levak.[5] The husband becomes his young wife's protector, and moreover he is thought to be the one who is responsible for her sexual development, according to Levak. The Bororos believe that menstruation cannot take place before the first intercourse and a man prepares his wife for this event digitally. The handling of her genitals is also thought to be the reason for the development of her breasts. For the Bororos, the husband is in charge of his wife's sexual maturation.

Among the Badaga of South India, homosexual relations occur between young men and boys as reported by Paul Hocking.[6] Lesbian relations are also presumed to occur, but Hocking says the only evidence for this is the belief of some informants that lesbian breast sex causes abnormally rapid growth of an adolescent's breasts, as seen in some girls.

When she is still small, a girl of the Aranda of Australia is promised to a man about the age of her father according to Geza Roheim.[7] However, the couple will not have intercourse until signs of puberty are evident in her. These signs according to Roheim are the development of her breasts and her pubic hair, and, of minor importance, the occurrence of first menses. In an initiation ceremony, as noted earlier, magical means are used to make the bride's breasts grow. Roheim adds that her intended husband then continues to visit the girl every so often to grease her and caress her, both of which are known ways to cause her breasts to develop and to show his love for her.

9

The start of a girl's sexual life

THERE IS WIDESPREAD CULTURAL correlation between the maturation of a girl's breasts and the onset of her sexual relations. This should not come as a surprise, for we know from this study that there is extensive use of the human breast as a means of obtaining sexual pleasure. However, the situation is mixed, because while in some cultures, sexual relations begin with the first development of the breasts, in other cultures sexual relations start at the first appearance of the menses. For the San of The African Kalahari Desert, both physiological processes are important. With the budding of her breasts, a girl begins a sexual initiation period, and with first menstruation, the initiation period culminates in a puberty ceremony. *The Biology of the San* by Ronald Singer is most informative on this topic.[1]

The !Kung and the G/wi are related language groups of the San people. A girl of the G/wi San is married at about seven or eight years old to a man who is perhaps seven years her senior, but sexual intercourse does not begin until early puberty, at the time when her breasts begin to develop. This was reported by Singer in the book mentioned above. Singer says that menarche, or first menstruation starts after about thirteen years of age, which is later than breast development. A. Stewart Truswell and John D. L. Hansen put first menstruation for the !Kung at 15 years.[2]

George B. Silberbauer says of the G/wi, that the marriage of a couple is without ceremony, marked only by the beginning of life together in a shelter.[3] This is later followed by intercourse when the wife's breasts develop, and then a ceremonial marking of puberty when she first menstruates. On this latter occasion the couple is symbolically joined and given advice concerning how to have a happy marriage. Menstruation is celebrated and regarded not only as the entrance into full womanhood for the female, but also as the finalizing of a couple's marriage.

Although !Kung San men and women are extremely modest about exposing their genitals, according to Lorna Marshall, a woman's breasts are left bare to nurse.[4] Modesty of behavior precludes the necessity for covering the breasts. In explanation, Marshall notes that the !Kung act with extreme reserve even in dancing, because they are always in the presence of those with whom they share an incest taboo, and any show of sexuality would be wrong. In contrast, Marjorie Shostak comments on the interest that !Kung men take of the changes in an adolescent girl's body, obvious because her breasts are not covered, and how the men joke about wanting to run off with her when her breasts mature.[5]

For the Ashanti of Ghana puberty rites are performed after the onset of first menstruation. Peter Sarpong reports that in the case of early menses, before the breasts are mature, a girl is advised to refrain from intercourse, and must wait a variable amount of time before she is initiated, even up to several years.[6] He says that an important factor in the delay is the state of the breasts, which must be firm and somewhat protruding. During these rites, the Ashanti remove a girl's clothes. Sapong relates that this is done so that people can witness that she has come of age, that she is not pregnant, and not of loose morality, which is indicated by the condition of her breasts.

For instance, pronounced drooping breasts are said to indicate pre-puberty sexual intercourse.

The Azande of the Congo calculate the sexual maturity of a girl by her breasts. E. E. Evans-Pritchard illustrates this fact by telling of Ngbiara, who, when her breasts matured, experienced intercourse with Bazingbi, a story that typifies young Azande sexual life.[7] According to Evans-Pritchard, the Azande believe that until a girl's breasts are formed, her mucus does not contain the souls of children; therefore a girl who has intercourse is not expected to become pregnant, and a young wife who does not give birth is not considered barren till after her breasts mature.

Among the Dogon of West Africa, marriage is arranged for the time when the breasts are formed, according to Genevieve Calame-Griaule.[8] At this time a girl has an ornamental nose ring inserted, although it is sometimes placed earlier when the girl is less fearful. The first intercourse must take place before a girl menstruates, because the blood of defloration is considered good blood, and must be distinguished from menstrual blood. Calame-Griule reports that a strict watch is kept on the development of the girl's breasts, which are the first signs of sexual maturity.

John Roscoe tells us that for the Ganda of Uganda, a girl's sexual maturity is gauged by observing whether or not her breasts bulge.[9] At about age twelve a girl shows signs of having breasts, which when large enough to drop down somewhat, denote a fully grown woman. According to Roscoe, first menstruation is often referred to as the time of marriage, and the girl is called a bride; this is reminiscent of customs of the San people. However, Lucy Philip Mair relates that older women of the Ganda teach that a girl should marry earlier than the first menses, as soon as her breasts drop, to guard against wantonness, which is thought to be unavoidable if she is not married when her breasts mature.[10] In relation to this, a girl is unclothed as a child, except for a fiber ring around her waist, but when her breasts begin to develop at twelve she wears bark-cloth around her hips as described by Roscoe.

A Zulu girl accepts the amorous attentions of a boy when she is about 14 years of age, according to AbsolomVilakazi.[11] However, he notes that she is not considered marriageable till her breasts are fully developed, somewhere around the age of sixteen years. Eileen J. Krige tells us that after having just reached maturity, Zulu girls appear at ceremonies for the first time almost naked except for some ornamentation, and participants comment on the firmness of their bodies.[12] A girl who wears a vest to cover her breasts on these festive occasions is criticized for trying to hide the effects of wanton behavior. Her exposed body declares her virtue and inexperience.

Two other examples illustrate the trend on the African continent. To be marriageable, a Hausa girl of Nigeria must have reached the age when her breasts have grown, as reported by Mary Felice Smith.[13] If she is not of the appropriate age, as indicated by her breasts, marriage is postponed. Similarly, a girl of the Maasai of Kenya and East Africa is not promised to a suitor until close to the time of marriage, when her breasts begin to develop, according to Paul Spencer.[14]

Several consultants, asked by Charulal Mukherjea about the age when the Santal of India first experience sex, had differing opinions.[15] Some thought at about fourteen or fifteen years for boys, when they reach puberty; and from twelve to thirteen years for girls, when their breasts mature. However, the ages ranged from ten to seventeen years for boys; and from nine to fourteen years for girls.

The Lur of Iran living in Deh Koh say that young brides there become pregnant before menarche, causing them to believe that sexual maturity is independent of monthly menstruation, as related by Erika Friedl.[16] A possible reason for this is that at first ovulation the young woman becomes pregnant, and the first menstrual blood is not shed, but is used instead to maintain the pregnancy. In other respects, a girl is thought to be mature for a variety of reasons: when she is somewhat competent with household chores, when her arms and face start to fill out, and when her breasts start to grow. Friedl points out that this description is compatible with the lower limit for a girl's marriage age specified by the Quran, that is, nine years.

Among the Kapauku of New Guinea, when a girl's breasts start to grow in her thirteenth year, she is defined as marriageable, while after her first menstruation she is defined as fully marriageable according to Leopold Pospisil.[17] Because the onset of menstruation comes later than breast development, first menses sometimes occurs after a girl is married.

Cora DuBois relates that for girls of the Alor Island of Indonesia, the first sign that the breasts are swelling indicates the girl's readiness for sexual relations, although the girl may have been married earlier.[18] Because of the very early marriage of girls, DuBois comments on the socially less trying period of adolescence for girls compared to boys. She notes that among the Alorese the first menstruation is treated as irrelevant, and Alorese women regard menopause in a similarly casual manner. According to DuBois several consultants told her that they became pregnant before first menstruation. The reason for this, as proposed for the Lur, is that with the first ovulation the girl becomes pregnant, and so the first menstrual blood is not sloughed off or observed.

One final story about the importance of the breasts in a woman's sex life – and in a man's. Melville Jean Herskovits describes the thoughts of a young man living in Dutch Guiana in South America, a descendent of escaped African slaves.[19] He begins to think about marrying a certain girl, but he knows that he has to wait until her breasts show, which by his reckoning might happen during the next planting. From this point, he is resigned to wait one or two months more before she will be ready to marry. His impatience and desire illustrate a phenomenon found in cultures around the world: the man waits for the woman's readiness for sex, that is, until her breasts have matured.

10

The breasts and clothing

THE EMERGENCE OF THE breasts signifies a young woman's readiness for sexual relations but also her future maternal role, presenting a dilemma as to how the breasts should be regarded. One function, the sexual one, does not exist among other mammals, and for humans it can be associated with guilty pleasure. On the other hand, maternal breast-feeding is righteous; it is ubiquitous among mammals, and necessary for mammalian life, except for humans who may substitute the bottle feeding of formula. The two differing purposes of the breasts are reflected in the conflicting requirements for non-exposure and exposure, and there are varied customs dealing with covering and uncovering the breasts. These customs are enmeshed with taboos concerning sexual behavior and the viewing of women's breasts. This is so because whereas human breast-feeding epitomizes love and can be openly performed, the breast sex of cultural sexuality, while also in the sphere of love, engenders envy and jealous reaction, and its performance must be hidden. In cultures where the breasts are uncovered during the day for nursing, there may be taboos preventing certain men from looking at them, usually relatives with whom sexual relations are forbidden. This does not stop other men from looking at them, but since nursing is such a basic, virtuous, and until recently, omnipresent activity, breast feeding considerations naturally take precedence over sexual considerations. Thus the woman engrossed in feeding her baby is not thought to be displaying her breasts in a sexual way for sexual purposes, as might happen at a dance, and staring by men is not expected.

The solution to the problem of the two meanings of the breast is succinctly summed up by William Kester Barnett, in the case of the Hokkien culture of Taiwan.[1] There, it is understood that despite the fact that the breast is a known object of sexual play, there is no immodesty on the part of a woman in breast feeding her baby in public.

On the island of Celebes in Indonesia, a young woman of the East Torajan culture hides her breasts from the sight of men, always keeping her upper body covered with a basic garment as described by Nicolaus Adriani.[2] The lower edge of the garment may be turned up to let air in but not so far as to be revealing, and a nursing mother will raise the garment above her breasts to nurse her child. To carry a load, a girl or young woman wears a head-cloth that spreads over her breasts and ties in the back. The clothing customs of the East Torajans demonstrate how the two functions of the breasts, the sexual and the nutritive, must be accommodated.

In the Tongan group of islands in the South Pacific, the code of dress promulgated by the 1850 Code of Laws required women to cover their breasts, engendering strict standards of modesty especially for adolescents. Commenting on this, Helen Morton Lee states that in pre-Christian times women did not cover their breasts unless they were pregnant or lactating, and even in more recent times older women sometimes leave their breasts uncovered without shame.[3] Gerd Koch mentions that in the villages of some of the islands, women and girls still worked in their huts with bared breasts.[4] This was in 1979. Exposed breasts were deemed tempting and shameful by early missionaries according to Christine Ward Gailey.[5] She termed this an assault on Tongan sexuality by the Wesleyan Methodists.

The transition from girlhood to adolescence is typically marked by a clothing change. Audrey Isabel Richards tells the story of two candidates at a puberty ceremony of the Bemba of Zambia, Africa, who while waiting at the initiation hut, had arranged their clothes to cover their breasts, as is the usual custom of Bemba women.[6] They were reprimanded and made to remove the covering from their breasts because their status as initiates was a lowly one.

Among the Saramaka of Dutch Guiana in South America the development of a girl's breasts is the traditional sign of readiness for the rites of womanhood as related by Sally Price.[7] When a girl's breasts are described as having dropped to the area of the heart she is ready to pass from adolescent aprons to the skirts of an adult woman according to Price. If an adolescent girl who is wearing aprons becomes pregnant she is immediately given skirts and married, and even without becoming pregnant she is given skirts if she is sexually active.

A girl of the Rungus Dusun of Borneo will start to wear a sarong at about the age of ten, slightly before her breasts begin to develop, and she is referred to as a sarong wearer, as described by Laura Appell.[8] As soon as breast development becomes apparent she is identified as a maiden, and she keeps this appellation until she is contracted for marriage. The author finds it important to emphasize that menarche, the onset of menstruation, does not constitute the start of a labeled stage in a girl's development in the Rungus Dusun culture. The appearance of breasts seems to be of greater importance.

While clothes and body adornment convey information about the sex, age, and status of the wearer, they also impart other social information. Special ornamentation of the breasts is used at festive events to make the wearer more sexually attractive, for instance the painting done by Tukano women of South America in preparation for a dance.[9] The wearing of beads and pendants appears to be ubiquitous as a way to accent the breasts. Even a gold cross around the neck can be used in an enticing way as seen in Ethiopia.

In the United States, different degrees of breast exposure depend on the occasion, place, and time of day – as well as the year or era. At times low décolletage is identified with evening wear, at other times it is fashionable for day wear as well. In the past, corsets have simultaneously cinched the waist and pushed up the breasts, or alternatively the flat look has predominated, as in the 1920s. Clothing customs are ever varying, with changes often influenced by clothing manufacturers. In the 1960s and 70s, the clothing of the "counter-culture" swept the fashion scene, led by the tastes of young people protesting war and sexual repression. "Love beads" were especially popular for both men and women, emphasizing the breast as the source of love.

11

The breasts in the cultures of the world: summary

IF BREAST SEX IS an important cultural phenomenon, we would expect to have this confirmed by anthropologists studying diverse cultures; specifically, we would expect descriptions of the breast in courtship, foreplay, and coitus. This has been confirmed, and more. Observations have shown that the breast occupies a place in literature, myth, humor, law, and ritual. Significantly breast sex can be identified with the sexual desire of the human female.

The male finds excitement in the form of the female breast: it denotes the woman's maturity and her sexual readiness. But there are consequences and taboos associated with this allure. Touching the breast is an act of seduction, implying an appeal to sexuality – an enticement to sexual intercourse. A man touches the breast of a woman to arouse her desire. As a preliminary sexual advance, this is seen in diverse societies, for instance at community gatherings such as at dances where the young can engage in sexual adventure. It happens in Alor Island in Melanesia and among the Santals of India, with the Tukano and Cubeo Indians of South America, and among the Lepchas of Sikkim.

The breast in various societies is covered by laws or prohibitions. Thus we see laws governing the treatment of the breast in the Kapauku culture of Papua New Guinea, among the Santal of India, and in the Rungus Dusun culture of Borneo where it is clear that touching the breast under circumstances where it is deemed a sexual transgression demands compensation to the victim or her family. In Kapauku society if the girl complains about an attempted seduction, it must be paid for, whereas in certain casual joking situations men may touch the breasts of women.

As for descriptions of the breast in foreplay and coitus – there are examples from various areas of the world. In Dogon culture, rape is referred to metaphorically as "cutting the breast", the opposite of sexual breast love. Among the Santals caressing the breasts is described as part of foreplay, and during coitus the man uses his hands on the breast to excite the woman. Among the Aranda of Australia a woman makes known her desire for sex by positioning her breasts against the man. In Chuuk culture, during intercourse, the man mouths the woman's breasts to enable climax. Among the Indians of the Sierra Nevada, the term "eating the woman" is used to denote cultural sexuality, implying among other acts, oral stimulation of the breasts.

The information gathered here reveals the daily sexual activities of human societies where the breast is vital to culture. The unique nature of breast sex is attested to by its absence in the sexual behavior of mammals other than humans. The various customs and laws that govern seeing, touching, and referring to the breast reinforce the idea that the breasts have great cultural and sexual significance around the world.

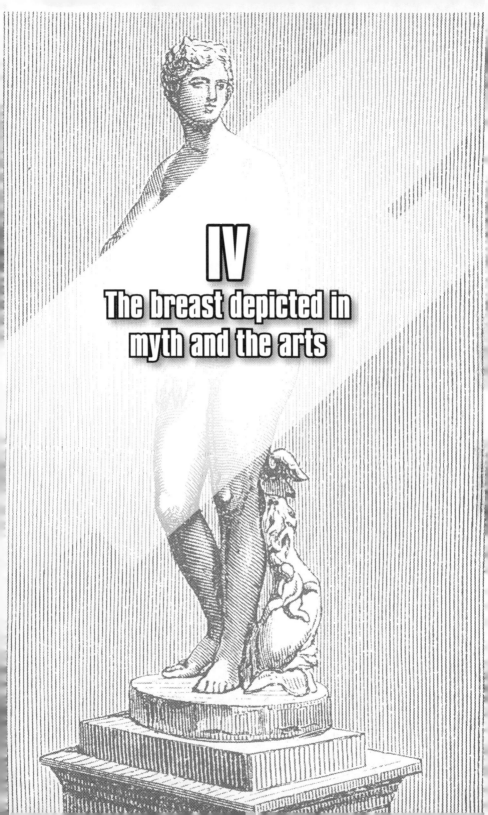

IV
The breast depicted in myth and the arts

1

Three creation myths

Ethiopia

A literary text of the Amharic people of Ethiopia concerns a prophetic dream about the transformation of Amharic culture brought about by Telahun and his wife Sophia. The dream reveals much about the sexuality of the people, and the centrality of the female breast in the transformation of their culture. In the dream, Telahun, grows a breast on his left side which embarrasses him and which he tries to hide. But he loves it so much that he kisses it and suckles it. To avoid jealous men who try to cut off his unusual appendage, he flees to the top of a mountain. However, on the mountain top when he tries to fondle the breast it is no longer there, and in its place is a beautiful young woman – his sister Sophia. In the given interpretation, Telahun attempts to hide Sophia and his love for her breast because they are brother and sister and they must marry in secret. According to the prophetic dream, in the darkness that covers the mountain, the epic couple open their mouths and light shines out, illuminating their entire environment, and by their example they improve the culture of the Amharic people. This story appears in *Dreams in Amharic Prose Fiction* by Taye Assefa.[1] Because of its themes of the female breast, love, and marriage, and because it links breast sex with speech and its power to metaphorically illuminate the world, this folk tale is about the transformation to cultural sexuality and to modern human life, with all that that implies, such as command of communication. It is also, strikingly, a variant of the story of Adam and Eve, as discussed below.

Judeo/Christian tradition

In the Judeo/Christian Biblical version of the Ethiopian story, Adam's significant appendage is a rib from which Eve springs-- thus she is his twin sister.[2] The breasts are again potent, albeit through the use of metaphor: with the eating of the apple, which is clearly Eve's breast, the couple gain knowledge of good and evil. God had commanded Adam not to partake of the fruit of knowledge – not to go beyond nature. When Adam disobeyed and God asks him why he did so, Adam responds that Eve offered the apple to him, blaming the woman as instigator. Eve, in turn, implicates the snake, the symbol of male sexuality and also of incest. In this Judeo/Christian version of cultural sexuality, the two commit a transgression against God and nature, and are banished from the Garden of Eden; they have forever left the ideal natural state and will suffer punishment forever. The wrathful Biblical God eventually supplants the local gods and goddesses of nature and of everyday human behavior, such as Astarte, the popular Canaanite goddess of sex and love. This negative assessment of breast sex and cultural sexuality is very different from that of the Ethiopian story above, and presages the medieval Christian negative attitude toward sexual pleasure and the female breast.

The Inuit of Canada

Intimations of sexual breast love can be found in the following story of a sister and brother, Seqineq and Aningat, the sun and the moon. It is one of the great Inuit myths, told in many versions. This is the Iglulik version, appearing in *Northern Voices*, edited by Penny

Petrone.[3] Aningat, who is blind and half starved by his grandmother, magically regains his eyesight, and so is able to see the evidence of his grandmother's cruelty to him. She had refused to let him have bear meat that she herself had been eating. Aided by his sister, Seqineq, he disobeys certain instructions of his grandmother, causing her death. The sister and brother then depart from their home and go out into the world. They settle among people who have no openings in the lower part of their bodies. When Seqineq delivers her own healthy baby, the other women become knowledgeable for the first time about sex, and cut slits in the appropriate places for intercourse and childbirth. When he desires intercourse, Aningat visits his sister only at night, putting out the lamp to keep her from recognizing him. But Seqineq marks Aningat with soot. When she finds that her brother is her unknown lover she cuts off one of her breasts and throws it to him, telling him to "eat it" because of his great fondness for her body. Aningat and Sequineq pursue each other outside the igloo, and as they circle around the igloo they rise into the sky: the sister, Seqineq, carrying a torch, is the sun, and her brother Aningat is the moon. This story contains elements of the other great stories of creation from Ethiopia, and from the Bible: forbidden food, leaving home after a transgression, incest, the potent breast (or apple), and the acquisition of knowledge.

2

Stories from around the globe

Greece and Somalia

Myth, folk tales, song, painting, sculpture, poetry and literature can elucidate the nature of cultural sexuality by description or absence of description. For instance, a wood carving of the marriage of the mythical Greek god Zeus and goddess Hera from the 7th century BCE, illustrates the significance of the breast in marriage for the ancient Greeks. See Figure 3.

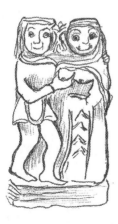

Figure 3
The sacred marriage of Hera and Zeus, wood carving; c. late seventh century BCE. Possibly from Samos. Drawing by the author from a photo courtesy of Deutsches Archaeologischas Institut, Athens.

However diffidence about sexuality shows its influence in the more recent personal folk songs of Greece according to Dorothy Demetracopulou Lee.[1] Very little of the body's anatomy is mentioned in love songs from this country, particularly sexual areas such as the female breast, says Lee. In 400 love couplets that she looked at only one mention is made of the female breast, in which it is likened to paradise. On the other hand, according to Lee, the term for the chest that pertains to both men and women is used freely, and the special term for the nursing breast is used regularly because there is no shame in exposing a breast to suckle a baby.

In the Somali culture of Africa, language subtleties and skills are greatly valued and discussed. Enrico Cerulli describes a Somali story about a camel driver visiting the city of Mogadishu who jokingly argues with a person from another tribe about the subtle meanings conveyed by their respective ways of speaking.[2] For instance, in one dialect if you say, regarding a man's wife that the man sucks the breasts of the one he sleeps with, it is translated in the other dialect into something that means the man sleeps with his mother. According to Cerulli, the description conveyed in the first instance is of a common occurrence, while in the latter instance it is a description of a taboo act. This is an example of the often indirect way that one finds out about the characteristics of human sexuality.

The Ifugao of the Philippines

In one of several stories of sister and brother incest, this one from the Ifugao people of the Philippines, a brother and sister live with each other and eat together, but the brother sleeps at night in another part of the house. The sister, wanting proof of her lover, puts lime on her breasts and navel, and in the night when the brother secretly comes to lie with her, it rubs off onto his body. The next morning the sister sees the lime on him and questions him. He replies that he was the one who came to sleep with her because there were no other people with whom they could marry, and otherwise humans would not multiply. This myth was collected by Roy Franklin Barton, and illustrates the ubiquitous association of the breasts with human sexuality and marriage, and the frequent reference to incest in human beginnings.[3]

The Mayans of Central America

The apple as breast is found in another culture, far from the Middle East. The religion of the Maya, according to Robert Redfield, reinforces old Mayan ways by combining their traditional beliefs with Christian beliefs, inclusive of both a rain-god and a contemporary God.[4] A Mayan informant gave his personal account of creation to Alfonso Villa Rojas[5], in which Adam and Eve were the first humans, created to care for an apple named "Chief". However Adam and Eve succumbed to temptation and ate the apple. A piece of the apple stuck in Adam's throat and became a protrusion there, symbolizing the male sex organ. In Eve, a piece of the apple became her breasts, and another piece became her genitals. The two began to think of ways to use their new organs, and upon discovering sex, they lived in sin. This brought about procreation and the multiplication of humanity. The Mayan retelling of the story of creation interestingly mixes up the apple with breasts and genitals.

In Mayan myth, the association between the breasts, cultural sexuality, and marriage is found in the following tale. It is the story of a giant who broke the necks of cattle, and of the youth who slew him with the help of a maiden. It was set down by Allen F. Burns. [6] The youth was attracted to three doves who were able at will to turn themselves into maidens. When he was about to go into battle against the giant, the youth announced that if he had only a small glass of wine, a biscuit, and the breast of a maiden to suckle, he could then rip the giant in half. Each of the maidens promised him this, but only one did as he had asked, and thus the giant was slain. When the couple returned to the girl's home they were advised by her father that because she had given her breasts to the youth, the two must marry and set up house together. They did this and lived happily nearby, an ending with which we are familiar.

Snakes or worms figure prominently in several myths related to fertility. The Mayans of Central America have a legend about a snake,

Chay Can, who chases nursing women to suckle at their breasts while inserting its double tail into their noses. According to Robert Redfield, this act is thought to result in death for a woman.[7]

The Tukanos of the Amazon and the Guarani of Brazil

Gerardo Reichel-Dolmatoff[8] reports a variant of the Mayan snake story among the Tukanos of the Amazon, who believe that a snake-like caterpillar can reside in the vagina and will come out and suck the breasts of a girl if she avoids ritual coition.[8] These similar myths from the Mayans and the Tukanos, conjure up images of breast sex and cultural sexuality.

In a belief of the Guarani of Brazil, a snake coiled at a nursing woman's breast stands for a sin or evil thing that she is doing, and that seeing the snake can make her child cry and refuse to nurse. According to Egon Schaden and Lars-Peter Lewinsohn, the sight of the snake must be blocked in order for the child to take the breast.[9] The lesson appears to be that nursing a baby must take precedence over having sex, particularly breast sex.

The Hopi of North America

In North America, in the Hopi ritual of the water serpent or palulokong, which is performed with puppets, snakes suckle at the breast of a symbolic woman. This is described by Mischa Titiev.[10] At the beginning of the drama, which takes place in a kiva, or Hopi house, corn plants which appear to sprout from earth mounds are placed on the floor, and sandpiper bird figures move back and forth overhead. The snake puppets emerge from behind a screen and they writhe and shake to indicate dancing and embracing, according to Titiev. A male performer plays the part of Hahai'i, an ancestral woman, who feeds cornmeal to the snakes and offers her breast to each one. In the story, the snakes have done the planting of the corn, and at the end of the ritual, after the simulated suckling of Hahai'i's breasts, they harvest the corn, which is enacted by knocking it over.

In the Hopi water serpent performance, the male symbolism of the snake can hardly escape notice. Alexander M. Stephen and Elsie

W. C. Parsons make abundant reference to the Hopi snake men and their rituals.[11] Birds, or the sandpipers in the Hopi ritual, are ancient symbols of female sexuality. In the interpretation offered here, the writhing of the snakes, signifying sexual embracing, indicates and completes the reference to cultural sexuality featuring the breast of Hahai'i, who is the ancestral female progenitor of the Hopi.

The Aranda of Australia and the Iban of Borneo

There is another tale of the snake and the breast, a myth of the Aranda of Australia, which depicts a large water serpent, or kulaia, who lives in a waterhole, and pursues a woman named Breast. The story is related by Geza Roheim.[12] The kulaia has star-like eyes and he swallows women; but Breast blinds him. Thus she is able to escape the usual fate of being swallowed up. The significance of the blinding may be similar to the meaning found in the aphorism that "love is blind."

From the Iban of Borneo, there is the following story of watery denizens and unrequited love, recorded by Edwin H. Gomes.[13] Two girls were catching fish in the river and storing them in a fishing basket. A fish jumped up from one girl's basket and touched her breast with its tail. She laughed, and said to him that not even her lover would dare to touch her breast in such a manner. The other girl laughed as well, and subsequently a storm arose with thunder and lightning and both girls were turned to stone. Apparently, the fish felt sexually spurned by the girl who did not welcome him to her breast.

The Middle East and early Native American Culture

While recalling the Old Testament story of the serpent and apple, symbolizing male and female respectively, the image of the medical caduceus comes to mind. The caduceus, found in early Middle Eastern and Greek iconography, depicts one or two snakes encircling a rod or tree and reaching toward a sphere, arguably the breast or apple of biblical parlance. The wings in this interpretation represent a bird in flight-- the entire scene signifying sex, pleasure, and good health.

Of related interest is the great serpent mound of southern Ohio, a Native American earthwork. The mysterious 1,000 foot long, three foot high sinuous serpent has in its open mouth, an oval breast-like structure which at one time was part of a scorched rock altar. This effigy mound is thought by some experts to represent a mythical water serpent which can also be seen in other North American depictions from the time. It is reminiscent of the Aranda myth of the water serpent who pursued Breast woman, and the Hopi pageant of the snake-men who suckled the breast of Hahai'i.

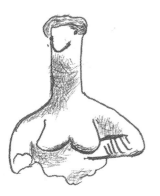

Figure 4
Bird/woman with arm supporting her breast; c. 5900 – 5700 BCE. Sesklo culture, (Megali Vrisi, Timavor), Thessaly. Drawing by the author after a photo from the Volos Museum.

In other symbolism concerning the breast, there exist paleolithic figurines from Europe, that are part bird and part woman and which exhibit prominent breasts. See Figure 4. Birds have long been associated with sex, fertility, and the family. The stork is known to children throughout northern Europe as the bringer of babies, and the goose is the emblem of family life and devotion to its mate, and is also associated with communication and story telling, as in "Mother Goose" tales. The bird-winged Greek sphinx, with a woman's head and rounded female breasts, is part beast as well – a lion sitting on its haunches. The sphinx is thought to symbolize the mystery of humanity.

Navaho and Western Apache of North America and the Bororo of Brazil

The Navaho tell the story of Be'gocidi, the son of the sun. This account is from Willard Williams Hill, and has an unusual emphasis on the breast and sex.[14] Be'gocidi was a mythic berdache, or homosexual, who could move about invisibly and who interfered with other people's sex lives. When a couple were engaged in intercourse Be'gocidi would run up, touch them, and shout "be'go, be'go", meaning "breast, breast"; or he would harasses hunters who had taken aim and were about to shoot, yelling "be'go, be'go" as he touched their testicles; and he would sneak up on young women and touch their breasts, all the while saying "be'go".

The Western Apache have a similar larger than life mythical character named Big Owl, who was known to do strange things as told by Grenville Goodwin.[15] He was looking for humans to eat one day, when he came up to a group of people who were camping. They recognized him and in fear they took off their clothes and claimed to have changed themselves into "ground heat". Big Owl checked out their claim by going up to all the women, feeling their breasts and between their legs. He agreed that they were ground heat.

Reminiscent of the western Apache myth is one from the Bororo of Brazil about first beings. The myth includes the story of a man identified as Bope, who was a very sexual being, and who retained many animal traits. The story is related by Zarko David Levak.[16] Bope had many wives and children and he liked especially to eat Bororo people. He preferred their sexual organs, that is, penises, vaginas, and breasts, which were procured for him by four of his warrior sons.

The Santals of India

The Santal's have a myth reported by William George Archer, that explains why women's nipples are black.[17] One day two Tudu boys who were iron-workers were making charcoal in the forest when they saw some bonga boys and girls approaching. The bongas were dancing, and the Tudu boys were afraid of the bongas' powers. The Tudus hid because they thought that they might die, but they were determined to dance with the bonga girls. They gave the girls flowers to smell and as a girl smelled a flower, a Tudu boy would confuse her by fondling her breasts. The Tudu's hands were black with charcoal and that is how women's nipples from then on were black.

The Aymara of the South American Andes

In folklore, hate, as well as of love, can be engendered by the breast: female demons from vastly different parts of the world are thought to have long hanging breasts. The Aymara of the South American Andes believe that certain demons, called japinunu, can seize people with their breasts, according to Alfred Metraux and Prisscilla Reynolds, and when the Aymara hear strange wings in the night, they know a japinunu is approaching.[18]

Palestine, Serbia, and Iran

In lore from the Middle East ghouls can be men or women; and the women have such long breasts that they can be flung back over their shoulders when moving, as reported by Hilma Natalia Granqvist.[19] These ghouls are said to be animals in the shape of humans, and they eat human flesh.

Serb peasants tell tales of fairies whom they claim can be seen both by day and by night according to Jeremija M. Pavlovic.[20] The fairies are said to be beautiful girls with long black hair who dance at night on the crossroads. One peasant told of seeing a fairy jump over a brook and as she jumped she tossed her breasts over her shoulders. He said that no harm came to him because he did not speak to her. Pavlovic recounts another story about fairies that tells of a man who found a baby in the forest and shaded the baby's eyes from the sun. A fairy appeared and asked who did the good deed and when the man answered, she gave him her breast to suck. Thus he achieved high status according to Pavlovic.

Among the Serbs, snakes are very much feared, and women are afraid that if they suckle a child of another ethnicity or religion, they will go to hell where their breasts will be sucked by snakes. Nevertheless, women will always suckle another baby when called upon in an emergency according to Milenko S. Filipovic, who gave this account.[21]

Similarly, as related by Henri Masse, many Iranian women are afraid to nurse a child of another religion for fear of ill effects.[22] These fears arise from a belief in the power of breastfeeding to confer siblinghood, a power as great as that of the uterus to do so. The idea that the breast can create siblings is also found in the Middle-east. In this respect, milk kinship is as potent as any other, and children who are breast fed by the same wet nurse may not marry each other.

The Azande of the Sudan, Africa

The Azande of the Southern Sudan say that a witch is fully conscious of his or her evil acts and leads a secret life, boasting and laughing with other witches about their ill deeds of hatred. Furthermore, the Azande believe that this hatred arises first in the breast and then descends to the belly, according to E. E. Evans-Pritchard.[23] The people say this explains a witch's consciousness. In another story from the Azande, related by Evans-Pritchard, a woman was seen suckling two kittens, one at each breast. The man who saw her had to go between her legs, and was sworn to secrecy or else the sight would be fatal to him.

The Garifuna of Honduras, Central America

Feminine spirits are thought by the Garifuna or Black Caribs of Honduras to tempt lonely young men who might be walking along a secluded path as recorded by Ruy Galvao de Andrade Coelho.[24] A spirit appears in the form of a beautiful young woman, one whom the man has loved, and when he follows her for some distance she reveals herself as an old hag with long pendulous breasts with which she lashes at his face.

The Sherpas of the Himalayas

An opposite scenario transpires in a fable of Tibetan Sherpas as told by Robert A. Paul.[25] In this tale a rock-demoness, in the form of a monkey, attempts to seduce a god with her vulgar motions, and when he refuses her, she is transformed into a beautiful woman who shows him her breasts and says that she desires him. She announces that they must set up house together, and that if he refuses her again, she will die and be reborn in hell. She further threatens to mate with an ogre and populate the world with ogres, perhaps a message for our time – that a return to the animal state and a world populated with barbarians is the alternative to woman's way of peaceful domesticity through our unique sexuality.

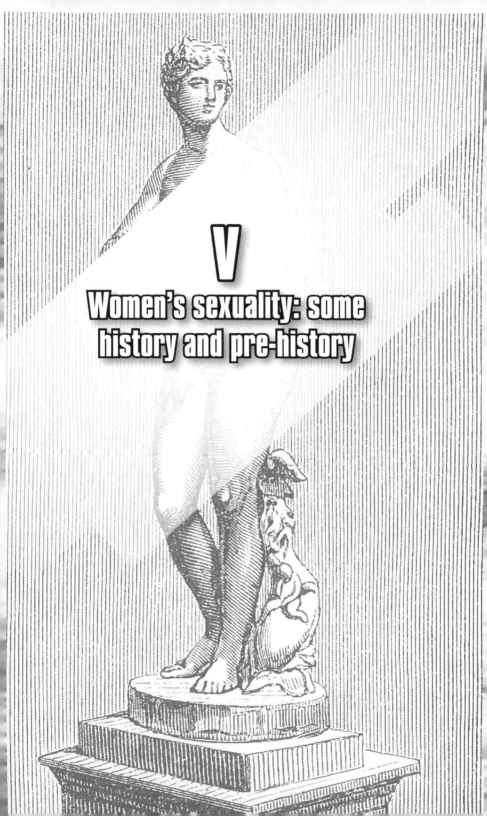

V
Women's sexuality: some history and pre-history

1

The breasts and religion

STARTING FROM THE STONE-AGE or Paleolithic period of some 30,000 years ago, a time when hunting was depicted on cave walls, small sculpted stone or ivory statuettes have been found in Europe that have been called deity images by some experts. Commentaries on the figurines take note of the female sexual aspect in these portable works of art. Sex, whether sacred or mundane, is suggested by the exaggerated breasts, buttocks and genitalia of the objects. Such statues were among the first indications of religion in early humanity according to Joseph Campbell, in his book, *The Masks of God: Primitive Mythology*.[1]

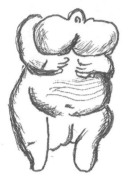

Figure 5
Venus of Hohle Fels; 38,000 -33,000 BCE. Swabian Jura, Southwest Germany. Drawing by the author after a photo from the University of Tuebingen, Germany.

So great is the purported beauty and voluptuousness of the small statues that they are sometimes called Venus figurines. The Venus of Hohle Fels from the European Stone-age of 38,000 BCE, only 2 1/2 inches high, was discovered by Nicolas J. Conard and his archaeological team in Germany and reveals in addition to her rounded body contours, two hands placed beneath her breasts.[2] See Figure 5. This placement can be compared with that in a later European statue, the bird/woman of 5900 BCE, addressed in the book *The Language of the Goddess* by archeologist Marija Gimbutas.[3] See Figure 4. Of interest, the bird/woman's left arm is held just below the prominent breast, as if displaying it. In certain Paleolithic and later goddess statues, until after the period of classical antiquity, a continuity of gesture can be discerned – the arms and hands framing and accentuating the breasts, making them a focus of attention. No infant is present in this statuary, suggesting that the purpose of the art is to depict the sexual use of the breasts. Additional relevant pre-historic statuary, such as the curvaceous Venus of Willendorf, whose arms rest gently just above her breasts, is treated more fully in *The Myth of the Goddess: Evolution of an Image* by Baring and Cashford.[4]

Some of the smallest figurines are female torso only, and in place of the head is a tab with a hole, as in the Venus of Hohle Fels, perhaps used for hanging the object on the body as a good luck amulet. In thinking about the purpose of the Stone-age figurines, research concerning extant hunter-gatherer groups is instructive. As told by Marion McCreedy, an anthropologist who worked with the

Biaka people of the Central African Republic, a notably egalitarian group, women are called upon to conduct rituals to increase the luck of hunters during times of hunting failure.[5] She goes on to describe other contemporary hunter-gatherers, for instance the Inupiaq of Alaska, and the Baka of Southern Cameroon, for whom women are considered to be mediators between the forest and the human world and who have the power to ritually call animals to the hunter. For similar reasons, Stone-age people, acknowledging the special qualities of women, including their unique sexuality, may have been inspired to carve female statuettes that were carried or worn around the neck by hunters to increase their chances of success.

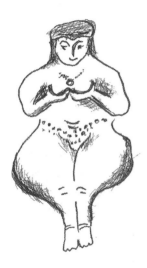

Figure 6
Ishtar, goddess of sex and fertility; c. 2000 BCE. Babylonian. Drawing by author after a photo from the Louvre (Art Resource).

Twenty thousand years after the European Stone-age, but with similar body language, female figurines from the Bronze-age of the Middle-east exhibit a characteristic stance associated with female deities of that time, known as the breast offering pose – a display of the breasts, lifted by arms or hands. Babylonian Ishtar, an icon of sex and fertility from 2,000 BCE, beckons with just such a pose in Baring and Cashford's book.[6] See Figure 6.

Ancient Sumerian writing and archeological items confirm that in the Middle-east cultural sexuality was once an aspect of various religions. These religions were populated with personified representations of natural and cultural phenomena, the goddesses and gods of the time. The acceptance of the sexual as sacred characterized the religions of the Bronze-age from about 3,000 to 1,000 BCE, and this approach lingered on in the polytheistic religions of Greece and Rome, up until the seventh century. After that, the priests of patriarchal religions, whose followers worshiped and committed themselves to one personal, mystical God, purged the veneration of the former gods and goddesses.

From the Bronze-age period of both bronze and clay objects, clay statuettes were found standing in many houses throughout the area of Canaan (present day Israel/Palestine), as revealed by archaeological excavation.[7] The numerous household statuettes, whether representing the female inhabitant of the house, or the local goddess, Astarte, as shown in Baring and Cashford, with hands or arms promoting her breasts, suggest that breast sex was deeply inculcated in the population.[8] See Figure 7. Just as some of the earlier Paleolithic European statuettes may have served as magical charms, so the Middle-eastern household figurines may have been the center of small shrines, thought to enhance fertility, sexuality, and domesticity, and to insure good luck in the harvest or in other endeavors.

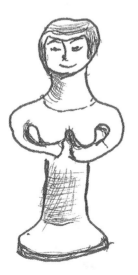

Figure 7
Astarte, Caananite goddess, unglazed earthenware; seventh century BCE. Tell Duweir, Israel/Palestine. Drawing by the author after a photo from the Metropolitan Museum of Art, New York (Art Resource).

The breast takes prominence in a portrayal, from the seventh century BCE, of the sacred marriage of the deities, Hera and Zeus.[9] See Figure 3. This brother and sister of the Greek pantheon of gods reveal in gesture and attitude, the promise of marital sex: Zeus holds Hera's breast in his hand, signifying the confirmation of their union. Again, from about 2,000 BCE, in a rendition of a marriage bed, the sexual suggestion of the breast is depicted in a clay plaque.[10] See Figure 2. Here, the wife holds her hand beneath her breast, seemingly about to offer it to her husband. In these scenes of intimacy, the potency of the female breast in the domestic realm is unmistakable.

In ancient representations of sex, the snake, signifying the male principle, often accompanies a goddess who, in one of the most revealing of these portrayals, is depicted sexually enmeshed with a snake in Baring and Cashford's book.[11] The art is thought to be Gallo-Roman, from the early centuries CE. The snake as phallus, appears to probe the vulva of the goddess with his tail, and at the same time he mouths her breast. An alternate interpretation says that she is giving birth to the snake, but the phallic symbolism is persuasive.

The island of Crete is another source of snake goddess imagery. Bronze-age writing of the Minoan people is not fully decipherable, and much knowledge of the culture comes from the art of the period, particularly from the palace of Knossos. Art work found there indicates the high status of women, who are often portrayed as athletes and priestesses. The frequent attire of the women of Crete, as shown in the art of the time, is a long dress with bare bodice, allowing exposed breasts. Goddess figures of the island are seen in several stances with snakes – handling snakes, draped with snakes, arms entwined with snakes -- signifying the sexuality and power of the goddess.

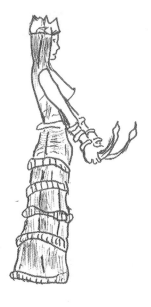

Figure 8
Gold-and-ivory snake goddess; c. 1500 – 1600 BCE. Minoan (Crete). Drawing by the author from a photo courtesy of the Museum of Fine Arts, Boston.

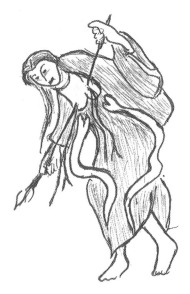

Figure 9
Woman representing Lust pierces breasts. Church fresco; early twelfth century, CE. Tavant, France. Drawing by the author from a photo in Marilyn Yalom, A History of the Breast.

Just such a Minoan female figure from around 1500 BCE in Crete contrasts with a female image from the middle-ages in France.[12] The difference in era is significant because by the medieval twelfth century, deities of the ancient world had been disinherited. The regal goddess of Crete is impressive in her posture which suggests her prowess and stature. Two snakes, worn like bracelets, stretch up from her extended arms as if searching for her breasts, one breast enticing with a golden knob for a nipple. See Figure 8.

On the other hand, in the Church fresco, an icon of Lust from twelfth century France, with symbolism similar to that of the Minoan figurine – breasts representing female sexuality and snakes as the male principle – offers a different version of religion: a rejection of the female body rather than its celebration.[13] Snakes leap up from Lust's legs, ready to attach to her breasts, but she prevents them from this act. Rather she pierces both breasts with a long spear and is depicted as cringing in reaction – her femininity negated, her sensuality denied. See Figure 9. Two contrasting religious views of womanhood are thus summed up: an affirming one that prevailed in the ancient world, a negative one in later times. In contrast to the extinguished beliefs of ancient Egypt, the Middle-east, Crete, Greece, and Rome, abnegation of the flesh, especially for females, is a recurrent theme of Christianity.

Up until about the seventh century of the middle-ages, women had deities to represent their interests, goddesses who were all too human and sexual in nature. For instance, Aphrodite and Venus were respectively the Greek and Roman goddesses of sexuality, love, and beauty. A statue called the Venus de' Medici, thought to be from the first century BC, emphasizes the breasts in a fashion similar to other goddess statuary: the fingers of one hand accent her breast, with an added feature – her other hand covers her genitals.[14] Cupid on a dolphin frolics at her feet. See Figure 10. Her pose, though subtle and apparently modest, links the breast to the genital sex act. Art informs about life in former eras, especially in the absence of the written word. With regard to women, we can observe two different religious views of the sexual breast: an ancient positive one versus a denial in later times.

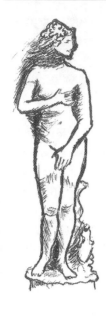

Figure 10
Venus de' Medici. Probably from
the first century BCE. Drawing by
the author from a photo courtesy
of Alinari Archives.

After the establishment of patriarchal religions, lingering participation in old religious rites, which might have included sexual acts, was inhibited by witch executions, culminating in the seventeenth and eighteenth centuries. The time of the New England witch trials was from the 1660s to the 1690s. In Europe the trials began earlier and ended later, the years of the major persecution being from 1560 to 1760. A primary cause, according to Elaine G. Breslaw, in the introduction to *Witches of the Atlantic World,* was the attempt to establish religious conformity in Europe and America.[15] A tactic was to rid the populace of domestic folkways that referred back to the beliefs and practices of ancient religions, including fortune telling, the casting of spells, and the making of folk medicine and love potions. The move to control domestic life fell hardest upon women. Women's sexual desire was deemed depraved by the Catholic church unless sanctified by marriage, and unmarried women, especially widows, were frequent victims of execution. Voltaire estimated that up to 100,000 witches were executed in the European hunts, perhaps 80 percent of whom were women.[16]

In the history of the persecution of women as witches, the female breast was thought to be especially susceptible to the devil. Protestant witch hunters of the Middle Ages claimed that nipples were sucked by the devil to gain power over women, and that nipples might be located in many parts of a woman's body. In writing about how witches were identified, Matthew Hopkins, in "The Discovery of Witches" in *Witches of the Atlantic World,* notes that a mark such as a wart or mole could be interpreted as a sinister "teat" used to nourish evil spirits, called familiars, and judged to be an indicator of a pact with the devil.[17] A common motif in the New England witch trials was the alleged observation of witches suckling these familiars.

The witch hunts in England and America were equaled in their zealousness by those in Germany and other countries of mainland Europe, in which religion reinforced class society and its corollary, male dominance. In Bavaria, Anna Papenheimer's breasts were cut off before she met her death by burning at the stake, as told in the book *Witchcraze by* Anne Barstow, who documents the terrible toll taken on women by an extreme methodology for keeping women in their place.[18]

An odious document, the Malleus Malificarum or Witch's Hammer of 1486, was used to incriminate women in cases of female barrenness, male impotence, failed births, the death of infants, and the destruction of crops and livestock.[19] This handbook, by the inquisitor priests, Heinrich Kramer (1430 to 1505) and Jacob Sprenger (from about 1436 to 1495) was well known in Europe and England, and was used as a guide in how to extract confessions of witchcraft prior to execution. From it we learn that procreation is a woman's duty, but that her sexual desire is excessive. Birth control and abortion are presented as never justified, and midwifery is maligned. The long arm of the Malleus Malificarum still has influence today over the domain of female sexuality, as women continue to wage political struggles to control our own bodies.

2

The uterus and medicine

FEMALE SEXUAL PHYSIOLOGY HAS been studied since ancient times, particularly the workings of the uterus. To understand women's sexuality, it is necessary to understand the physiology of the uterus, as well as of the breasts and genitals, because they function together. Plato writing from the 400s into the 300s BCE, made reference to the womb as a living thing, desiring union, which if not satisfied travels around the body causing havoc with various organs. Hippocrates, the man named as the father of modern medicine, writing at about the same time, also expounded on this idea of the "wandering womb" and its moisture seeking tendencies. These and other interesting facts concerning early attempts to characterize the uterus are explored by Helen King in her book, *Hippocrates' Woman, Reading the Female Body in Ancient Greece.*[1]

The perception that the uterus was sexual, although primitively envisioned, prevailed in ancient times. Hippocrates believed that the womb required moisture to maintain its health, and this idea contributed to his conviction that sexual intercourse was a treatment for uterine disorders. According to King, in the gynecological theories of Hippocrates, the dry womb was thought to turn this way and that in seeking moisture, and even to move to the liver, diaphragm, and other organs in its quest. When the uterus rose up in the abdomen, and turned or moved to various parts of the body, a professed effect was a feeling of suffocation for the woman. Hippocrates maintained that women affected by uterine symptoms were often those who abstained from or did not have intercourse, including virgins and widows, and his remedies often included sexual relations.

The survival of Hippocratic teachings continued on into the middle-ages through various translations of his work. King notes that the gynecological descriptions of the uterus by Hippocrates were used by later physicians in their delineation of the condition that came to be known as hysteria. The notion of the "wandering womb" was still widely accepted, whether as literal belief or metaphor for sexual desire. However, the physician, Galen, writing in the second century, although regarding sexual intercourse as therapeutic for so-called symptoms of hysteria such as feelings of suffocation, did not accept the idea of the wandering womb.

In the second century, when more was known about anatomy, the Greek physician Aretaeus, had an explanation for the womb's effect, as related by King, writing in the book *Hysteria Beyond Freud*.[2] Realizing that membranes prevented it from moving very far, Aretaeus thought the womb exerted its influence through contact, or sympathy, with other organs. In particular, he believed when the womb rose up and pressed on the intestines for a long time, the pressure was transferred to the diaphragm and lungs, and brought about loss of breath. Women themselves, particularly midwives, must have contributed to the thinking of the time. For instance, according to King, Galen relates the case of a woman widowed for many years who was told by a midwife that her symptoms were caused by a womb that was drawn up. Limited though their ideas were, we should not fault the ancients for attempting to understand the female body.

We know today that the uterus does rise in the abdomen. In their work in 1966, the researchers, Masters and Johnson determined by pelvic examination, that the non-pregnant uterus is capable of rising during sexual arousal in much the same say that the penis becomes erect.[3] They demonstrated that in response to sexual stimulation, the uterus elevates during both the excitement phase and the plateau phase. At the end of the plateau phase the uterus typically has increased in size by 50 to 100 percent, and they showed that after orgasm the uterus again returns to its resting state, reducing in size during the resolution phase.

In the diagnosis and treatment of disease, doctors of the middle ages continued to use the translated texts of Hippocrates and Galen, but authorities wishing to control the general populace, often named the devil as the cause of disease, and women were frequently identified as his agents. Woman's unique sexuality was debased and attacked. The Protestant church targeted women's breasts. The Catholic church targeted women's so called deficiencies in giving birth and at the same time censured their sexual passion. By the middle ages, a woman's opportunities to understand her body, instead of improving, were greatly diminished.

Toward the end of the nineteenth century the medical specialty of gynecology was born, and with it began the practice of removing women's reproductive organs in response to various diseases and complaints. Regina Morantz-Sanchez in her book *Conduct Unbecoming A Woman* documents these times.[4] The fact that in cases of diseased organs, surgery was necessary and beneficial does not excuse the excesses. Ovariotomy, a term used in the nineteenth century for elimination of the ovaries, was practiced for any number of reasons, including removal of healthy ovaries to cure the so-called hysterical syndrome. Morantz-Sanchez relates that routine pre-surgical biopsies were not yet the norm, and surgeons often foisted surgery without justification on women who sought help. Progress in surgical techniques demanded guinea pigs and women from the poor classes served this purpose well. Elizabeth Blackwell proposed to rally other women physicians against ovariotomy, and Mary Spink, also a physician, criticized male gynecologists for their primary role in ovariotomy excesses.

Removal of the uterus, or hysterectomy, was a dangerous procedure in the early days of female abdominal surgery and too risky to be performed regularly, but in the late 1880s surgeons learned to control the bleeding associated with hysterectomy. When a certain level of expertise in uterine removal was reached, ovariotomy declined in favor of hysterectomy, according to Morantz-Sanchez. Charges that such surgeries unsexed a woman were leveled right from the start, but the determination to ignore the sexual function of these organs was notable. At the time of consultation, physician explanations were rare of the after effects of surgery, for instance loss of sexual feeling and desire.

Although life threatening surgical effects can still arise today with hysterectomy, it is considered a safe procedure. For the treatment of cancer, doctors agree that the hysterectomy is a necessity. But for other conditions alternatives exist which may not always be used. So say William H. Parker, MD, and Rachel L. Parker in their book, *A Gynecologist's Second Opinion.*[5] Benign conditions for which hysterectomy is performed include uterine fibroids, endometriosis, heavy menstrual bleeding, and prolapsed uterus. In 2003, over 600,000 hysterectomies were performed in the United States, of which over 90% were for benign conditions.[6] This wasting of the uterus is a phenomenon of the U.S. more than anywhere else. In other countries the situation is different. In 1997 it was reported that in France the hysterectomy was almost never performed for fibroids, and in Sweden the rate of hysterectomy was one quarter that of the U.S.[7]

It may be true that women who suffer from various types of pelvic and lower back pain, and from prolapsed uterus, seek out and insist on surgery, but reactions to the outcome can vary. Some women say they are grateful for the operation that rids them of the bothersome uterus with its messy and sometimes painful functions; others have a very difficult time reorienting their lives after the hysterectomy.

Even with new surgical options, a question remains: do some 600,000 women a year really need to undergo high tech surgical procedures on their sex organs? If so, research into the poor state of women's reproductive and sexual health should begin immediately. For those contemplating this surgery, the HERS Foundation provides information and services related to the hysterectomy.[8]

The interaction of breasts, uterus, and genitals characterize the unique female sexual act, an act more complex than that of the male. But as different as the sexual behavior of the two sexes may be, there is a parallel occurrence in the male and female: the sexual response – the experience of orgasm. Interestingly, while it is generally known that the female clitoris is a homologue of the penis and performs an erotic function in the sexual arousal and climax of women, a little known fact is that the male prostate gland has imbedded in it a small homologue of the uterus, called the prostatic utricle.[9] Its exact function is unknown, but it is no doubt an erotic one, perhaps having to do with male orgasm.

Both uterus and prostate beat rhythmically during orgasm, in female and male respectively. Masters and Johnson demonstrated this in their study of human sexuality. Thus the prostate for the man, and the uterus for the women are locales of the human sexual response. If these organs are removed, sexual dysfunction is frequently reported. Despite benign conditions that affect it, the removal of the prostate is often avoided except in cases of localized cancer. The same care and concern for the quality of sexual life that men receive should be accorded to women in the performance of the hysterectomy.

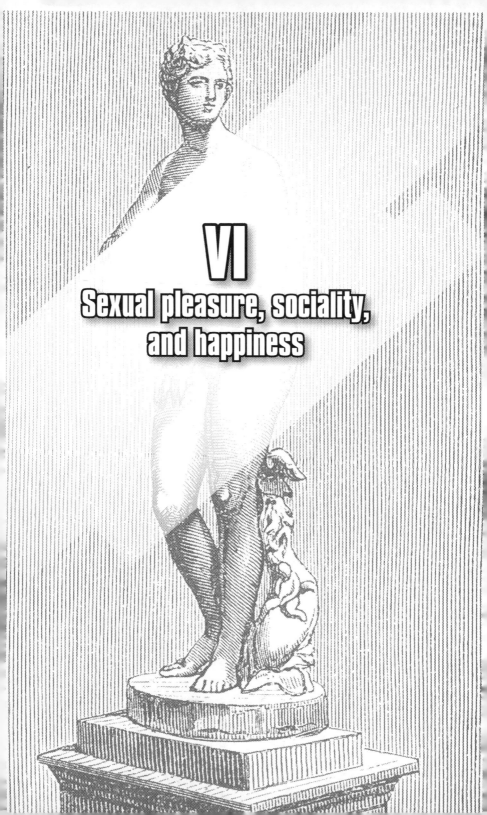

VI
Sexual pleasure, sociality, and happiness

1

Orgasm and equality between the sexes

THE QUESTION OF FEMALE orgasm in other primates is still in contention, but concerning a highly pleasurable version, there is some agreement that only in the modern human species do females experience this. The zoologist, Desmond Morris the author of *The Naked Ape*, in speaking of female monkeys in heat, notes that after copulation is completed, the female monkey continues on her way as if nothing much had happened, showing little indication of emotion.[1] This description of female monkeys applies equally well to both males and females of other nonhuman species after copulation, as seen in chimpanzees by Jane Goodall.[2] This does not mean that mammalian mates do not at times demonstrate affection for one another. The crux of the matter may be that for both male and female nonhuman primates, there is small capability for strong positive emotion, and this may have to do with the nature of their sexual experience – the absence of breast sex.

According to Morris, among the primates, human female orgasm is unique. However, orgasm has been inferred in nonhuman female primates by researchers like Goldfoot and co-workers, who noted uterine contractions and increased heart rate during genital sexual interactions;[3] and Burton, who saw reactions to experimental genital stimulation.[4] Some researchers have noticed a characteristic facial expression in these females during sexual contact, for instance Chevalier-Skolnikoff,[5] and also DeWaal.[6] Similar signs in male nonhuman primates, such as a fixed stare at the time of ejaculation, have been accepted as sufficient indications of pleasant sensations or orgasm, as noted by Pavelka.[7] In other indications, females will rub their genitals on objects in the environment until they produce an orgasm-like reaction according to Pavelka. The question might rest with the definition of orgasm, which in our own experience involves not only physical pleasure, but shared positive emotion, cognitive involvement, and cooperation between the partners. Then satisfaction can be profound and highly meaningful.

Although physiological indications of female orgasm have been detailed in monkeys and chimpanzees, the physician Leonard Shlain in commenting on this fact, notes that these expressions of orgasm in female nonhuman primates are feeble in comparison to those of woman.[8] Donald Symons concluded in 1979 that although the question of nonhuman female orgasm was still open there wasn't enough convincing verification of it.[9] However, as noted, researchers have presented evidence of physiological reactions to sexual contact indicating pleasure. If some sort of sexual pleasure, no matter how minimal, is experienced by nonhuman primates, then sexual pleasure must have been experienced by our earliest human ancestors.

Signs of pleasure in nonhuman primates have also been documented in contexts other than intercourse, for instance during masturbation, as seen by Pavelka, and this fact has significance for the present. As noted by Shere Hite in 2004, orgasm at the time of intercourse, although notably easy for men, is known to be relatively difficult for women, and women often masturbate as an accessory to sexual intercourse.[10] Early human females may have practiced self-induced sexual pleasure, especially around the time of estrus when the sex drive is greatest, and at other times as well. For bonobos, the practice of masturbation was shown in a study conducted by deWaal of bonobos or pygmy chimpanzees in captivity.[11] Of 39 masturbations observed by deWaal, about 23 percent of them were performed by the two adult females, none were performed by the one adult male, 59 percent were performed by the two adolescent males, and the rest, or 18 percent, were by the juveniles of the study. But however pleasurable masturbation may be, it is arguably not as gratifying as intimate sexual options between partners, as Abramson and Pinkerton suggest in *With Pleasure: Thoughts on the Nature of Human Sexuality.*[12] That is, relational sex, or interpersonal sex, rather than going it alone, makes for a more meaningful experience.

In nonhuman primates, in addition to male-female sex, same sex relations have been widely observed, and have been thoroughly documented in bonobos by deWaal.[13] The bonobo repertoire of non-reproductive sex, including masturbation and same sex genital rubbing, serves to reduce tensions, allowing bonobos to associate more easily, according to deWaal. There probably was a similar effect of non-reproductive sexuality among early humans that allowed a weakening in dominance relations and greater association between members of a group. In a milieu of varied reproductive and non-reproductive sex, females had the flexibility to discover the sexual potential of the breast. The sexual equality that ensued challenged any remaining authority of dominant males.

Our intense human sexual life and its several complements— sexual equality between a relating couple, love, the pair-bond, and cooperation in family and multi-family surroundings – set us apart from the other primates, notwithstanding many similarities to them. At some point in time, 7 to 8 million years ago, we and chimpanzees shared a common ancestor. Later, a species in the human line, *Australopithecus*, from 4 or 5 million years ago, took the significant step of walking upright, but in some respects it was not far removed from apish ancestors. Several human species arose and went extinct in the course of human evolution. At around 1.8 million years ago, *Homo erectus*, with bigger brains and the ability to relate to more conspecifics, emerged, and remained till about 250,000 years ago. That is a time when our present species,

Homo sapiens, or anatomically modern humans is thought to have emerged. *Homo sapiens* can be characterized by the sexual breast and cultural sexuality, but this way of sexually relating may have first showed glimmerings of existence with an archaic form of *Homo sapiens* some 300,000 years ago, becoming fully functional around 150,000 years ago. Perhaps, not coincidentally, this is when complex language may have been emerging. Philip Lieberman in his book, *Eve Spoke: Human Language and Human Evolution,* puts the appearance of fully developed language at about 150,000 years ago.[14] This is the point in prehistory, as conjectured here, that cultural sexuality with its important aspects of equal pleasure for a sexually relating man and woman began to shape our destiny and to influence cooperation and communication.

Christopher Boehm in his book, *Hierarchy in the Forest,* analyses egalitarianism and moral life in human society, especially as exemplified in the societies of hunter-gatherers.[15] He believes that humanity's cultural and behavioral readiness for egalitarianism was not reached until the time of anatomically modern humans, 100,000 years ago. His analysis is not about gender relations, but some of what he says is pertinent to the establishment of cultural sexuality, with its characteristic equality and cooperation between men and women, as seen among hunter-gatherers and in contrast to primate societies dominated by alpha males. Boehm feels that the attainment of general social egalitarianism was revolutionary because, "to eliminate the alpha role decisively, the rank and file may have needed to use force." This may also have been the case in the establishment of cultural sexuality as a way of life—male dominance had to be overcome.

It can be speculated that equality between men and women in the sexual sphere was necessary to the creation of a general state of social egalitarianism. The inauguration of sexual equality meant countering the dominance of anti-cultural powerful persons who nevertheless continue to exist today – not part of the mainstream of humanity, but the top ruling oligarchs. Referring to legend, the Inuit relate that a powerful shaman attempted to kill the inhabitants of a new colony founded by females on Southampton Island, but did not succeed, as described earlier in this text.

According to the Marxist anthropologist Eleanor Leacock in her book, *Myths of Male Dominance*, women in egalitarian hunter-gatherer societies were in the past socially equal to men, and it was only with the subsequent growth of private property and the repercussions of class society that this parity was lost.[16] She cites the journal of the Jesuit, Father Le Jeune, who lived with a group of Labrador natives, the Montagnais, in the winter of 1633-1634, in which the priest described the women as having "great power" and "choice" over the plans and undertakings of the band. The priest appeared however not to approve, and lectured the Montagnais men about the disobedience of their wives. Constant effort must be expended by women to obtain and maintain their rights, although the past establishment of cultural sexuality set the stage for woman's full social equality.

2

Cultural sexuality: positive emotions and sociality

ALTHOUGH CHANGES IN WOMEN'S sexuality have been thought to be important in evolutionary development, particularly by anthropologist Donald Symons,[1] the adoption of breast sexuality seems to have escaped consideration. It is suggested here however, that this new way of having sex – its initiation and spread – set off a big upheaval in the way the sexes acted toward one another, causing a change in basic human sociality. It enabled a common sexual ground of intimate pleasure and interdependency from which knowledge of the mental states of self and other and empathy could follow. It brought about commitment and devotion to one another from which the human family could spring. Humans became the ultimate mammals, using the mammary gland in a novel way that affected the brain as well as the sex organs, causing new emotions and new cognition.

The practice of sexual breast love or cultural sexuality embodies greater sociality of the human sexual pair as compared to non-human primates. The male and female, as never before in evolution, began to have intimate knowledge of each other's wants and needs. They communicated their desires through sound, gesture, and word and were able to reciprocate by fulfilling each other's sexual needs. Complementary caresses by male and female demanded coordination and cooperation, which brought about a ritual of satisfaction.

Furthermore, because of the greater passion and longer duration of the human sex act, people became more sensual. Increased tactile sexual play between a couple, engaging the whole body, but particularly the genitals and breast, was cultivated, accompanied by sexual arousal. With sexual arousal and sexual thoughts, as shown by J. Bancroft, oxytocin is implicated.[2] Sexual passion became possible at unforeseen moments, far from the time of biological heat or estrus, the monthly peak of primate female desire and desirability. Although it has been shown that chimps and especially bonobos have extended their sexuality somewhat beyond the confines of estrus, they are still tied to it, while men and women can become desirous of each other at any time – for instance even during menstruation.

The increase in pleasure and sociality in this sexual collaboration led to an increase in the positive emotions, such as love, pride, and happiness; and our exotic sexual practice spread. In a study of the transmission of positive emotions in 4,739 people over a twenty year time span, Nicholas Christakis and James H. Fowler found that when people changed from an unhappy state to a happy one, others in their social network became happier too.[3] Professor John Cacioppo, director of the University of Chicago's Center for Cognitive and Social Neuroscience believes that the study reflects an evolutionary trend to "select into circumstances that allow us to stay in a good mood."[4] In congregating together, people seek to learn the secret of happiness from each other. The smile, denoting sociability and happiness, is a hallmark of humanity. From the standpoint of cultural sexuality, communing with and learning from others allowed the practice of breast sex to spread and the happiness of sexual satisfaction to increase.

In human development, the advent of love and an increase in the positive emotions was fundamental. But an analysis of love presents problems because its relationship to sex can be misunderstood. The sociologist, Robin Allott who examined the evolution of love, says that the systematic treatment of love has been meager—a topic thought not to be serious, and not appropriate for scientific study.[5] Allott, in his investigation of love, brings in various strands. He implicates empathy, which has a cognitive component, as an important element of love, but he finds that acknowledging a role for empathy does not demonstrate how love evolved.

Allott sees the mother/infant bond as a candidate for the source of love, but he perceives the extension of love to others as solely a neural relation between people, not a bodily relation, and he does not consider sexuality as being instrumental in the evolution of love. He hesitates at this idea, noting that among non-human animals the connection between sex and love is non-existent; he says that there is no precedent for love to proceed from sex. This is a dilemma unless one accepts the idea that human sexuality is cultural and thus different from non-human sexuality. While still remaining creatures of nature, people were able to move into the realm of modern culture.

The answer to the question posed by Allott of how sex and love are connected is found by acknowledging humanity's conscious intention to practice sexual breast love. Mammalian sexuality is understood to be primarily instinctual, or an unconscious drive, but humanity's sexual breast love originated in a voluntary and deliberate way, and subsequently came to be learned in the community. What did women want of sex, and what do they still want? It is said that women crave love, but love cannot be divided from the shared relationship that accompanies it; in addition to the physical pleasure, women desire an enhanced social bond. The philosopher, Herbert Spencer in his sociological exposition, *Social Statics,* examines the idea of human happiness. In his analysis, the human strategy to obtain greater happiness is to become more social and in so doing "fulfill all human desires."[6]

Sociality is a crucial added dimension in cultural sexuality. By means of cultural sexuality women not only experienced greater pleasure, but began to extend to the engaged male, the love and intimacy that were formerly extended only to offspring. In return, it became possible for women to receive similar love from men. More time was spent in intimate bodily interaction, providing the common ground from which to recognize the other's feelings and thoughts, that is, to appreciate and empathize with the other and to bring about a new inter-gender social organization.

Thomas Gregor is an anthropologist who writes about sexuality and love. He observes with surprise the extent to which sex is portrayed in scientific texts as if detached from the positive emotions.[7] He notes that while it is clear that sex can take place without love, on the other hand, not love without sex. According to Gregor, sex is the "cornerstone" of love as well as of its various aspects such as affection and commitment; however, he says that the current nature of our society is repressive, and therefore there is a lack of understanding of both sex and love. But even in repressive societies, loving relationships somehow flower as Gregor shows in the lives of the tribal Mehinaku people of Brazil.

Although love in some tribal societies is thought by some anthropologists not to exist or to be repressed, in a cultural study by W. R. Jankowiak and E. F. Fisher, they find that love is a human universal or near universal.[8] Since, as conjectured in this book, breast sex was the origin of love between the sexes, it may be, or was at one time, another near human universal.

3

Happiness and human development

WHERE DO POSITIVE EMOTIONS come from? Cultural sexuality of the breast is a good candidate for their substantial appearance, inspiring not only physiologically based love, but pride and joy in achieving sexual satisfaction and in forming successful relationships. The dawn of sexual breast love brought into being a completely new social situation for humanity and today its practice is likely to contribute to a happier, healthier sexual and emotional life.

Theodore Kemper, an expert on the sociology of emotions, tells us that as long as society gives rise to new social situations, new emotions continue to appear.[1] In his work, he finds that satisfaction is a primary emotion that is physiologically grounded, and that there are related secondary emotions, such as love, pride, and gratitude that people are socialized to experience.

Pride, joy, delight, and ecstasy are new emotions, not found in the chimpanzees, writes sociologist Jonathan Turner in his book *On the Origins of Human Emotions*.[2] Turner discusses the individualistic nature of the apes, and the low content of satisfaction and happiness in apes such as the chimpanzees despite the presence of the mother-infant bond. In contrast, in humans he notes that selection occurred for the positive emotions which are used in the building of social bonds. He says this was necessary to solve the problem of making humans responsive to each other and willing to cooperate.

The qualities of kindness and tenderness are named allies of love by Zoltan Kovecses in his book *Emotion Concepts.*[3] It may be added here that kindness and tenderness are often associated with the breast-- appropriate to the concept of sexual breast love that is being considered. Kovecses points out the connection between love and the positive emotion of happiness. He states that while intimacy and sexual desire are the antecedents of love, reciprocal love is the antecedent of happiness. It appears, in light of what is suggested in this book, that the reciprocal ways of cultural sexuality must precede happiness. To make a comparison: there is nothing mutual in the manner of chimpanzee sex, while the way of human sexual interaction is a gratifying give and take.

The distinguished social psychologist, Barbara Frederickson, has found that the love that people experience consists of many positive emotions, and she names joy, interest, and contentment.[4] She goes on to say that social bonds are built up through playful and satisfying interactions that are motivated by love, and that these social bonds in turn allow future love and help. In a long view of human personal relations, it appears that there is an alternating implementation process of love and social bonds.

Frederickson emphasizes the influence of the positive emotions on cognition. She characterizes the positive emotions, such as interest and contentment, as emotions that generate changes in cognitive activity, followed by possible changes in physical activity. She points out that circumstances that promote the positive emotions broaden people's attentional scope, allowing them to see the whole picture – the forest as well as the trees.

This broadening effect was looked at by Annette Bolte and her research team.[5] They demonstrated that in the brain, holistic information processing, which is concerned with the whole picture, is helped by an increase in the positive emotions. In their study of word association, they saw that, under the influence of a positive mind set, wide rather than narrow word associations are activated in the memory, including remote word connections. Further, they say that these extensive associative brain networks, set in motion by a positive mood, allow creative problem solving.

The philosopher, Herbert Spencer, who was noted for his psychological insight, saw a connection between sociality and happiness.[6] He also identified a connection between happiness and mental activity. In discussing the political right to a claim on life, he comments on people leaving the isolated state. He says that upon becoming more social, we obtain the security and happiness that give us the freedom to exercise our human faculties, that is, the mental and bodily powers that affect our consciousness. He was especially interested in the mental faculty of sympathy, or empathy, which enables morality. According to Spencer we voluntarily enter a state of greater sociality precisely to become happier, with all the advantages that follow.

Along with the exercise of greater cognition allowed by the positive emotions, modern humans are characterized by the usage of complex language in which the positive emotions, such as commitment, play a role. Commitment is a component of love, as analyzed by Robert Sternberg's in his triangular theory of love, and as such it is a positive emotion.[7] Commitment as an aspect of love is also commented on by Thomas Gregor.[8] Commitment is necessary for dialogue to take place according to linguistic anthropologist, William Hanks.[9] He says that the language and the talk of social life depend on background understandings gained in human interaction. He adds that to resolve meanings there must be mutual orientation, and importantly, that this mutual orientation "works through common ground, participatory commitments, and joint activities." It can be conjectured that in the general context of the commitment and common ground established through cultural sexuality, dialogue between the sexes might have first started with reference to the sex act, specifically around the demands by women for breast sex, and then was extended to other spheres of social life.

The passion of cultural sexuality enables the motivation and purpose necessary for people to gain significant knowledge of each other, starting with their own bodies. Mutual knowledge, or shared information provides a common ground or content from which people can work together. Herbert Clark and Susan Brennan say that common ground is the basis for the coordinated and synchronized action of many human activities, including lovemaking and conversation.[10] They note that people keep track of their common ground and its minute-to-minute changes in a process called grounding, which allows both collective action and communication.

Until the sexes began to interact in a reciprocal and mutual way there was probably no highly enhanced communication. With love, empathy, and sharing between adults, everything changed. The pair-bond and the family were able to evolve, and people became more cooperative with each other – and, significantly, more communicative. What we were able to accomplish with all this was modern language, which probably exists, at the most basic level, to facilitate sex, love, and the pair-bond.

This development was comparatively sudden, but it did not happen all at once. First of all there is a cost involved in rising to a new level of sociality, because, as most of us can attest to, it takes work to maintain a close relationship, let alone a society. With feminine motivation, humans chose increased sexiness and intimacy despite the increased work of sustaining love relationships and raising children. And it must have required some time for our ancestors to change from the promiscuous sexuality that characterizes the chimpanzees, and likely also our early ancestors, to the pair-bond that typifies today's basic love relationships. The pair-bond, based on cultural sexuality and love, together with the cooperation and work necessary to maintain love, is the foundation of our modern human culture.

With the adoption of sexual breast love and pair-bonding, the sexes for the first time began to reside together as couples within their communities. In this situation, men could be enlisted in the raising of children in families and in extended families. The sexes were able to cooperate in providing nutrition and the teaching of offspring, dividing the labor as needed to carry out this project. Thus males began to take responsibility for the survival of the next generation for the first time, relieving females of some of the burden.

4

Past and present

BREAST SEX WAS A significant practice in the past, as has been described in ethnographic accounts of mostly non-literate societies. Breast sex is still a significant practice today as shown for instance by Dr. Kinsey,[1] and in *The Hite Report*.[2] People introduced it at some time in our pre-history and it provided a new and unique social environment, one in which advanced human culture developed. The use of the breast for sexual gratification might be characterized as a kind of expertise that was instigated by our ancestors – a unique cultural practice, as also is speaking, for instance. By using the breast as a means for revolutionizing the human female sexual response, we brought about a new psychological state of love, and a higher form of behavior. We achieved the sociality of pair-bonding, cooperation, and advanced communication. This is the constellation of love.

Symbolically the breast signifies not only nurturance but sex. Exactly how our predecessors first recognized and promoted the sexual breast is not clear, but because its use in copulation was pleasurable for women, in a deeply social act, and because it promoted the pair-bond and happiness, mammary eroticism was adopted in ancient communities and the technique was passed from generation to generation. This involved repeated acts of will and energy to overcome reliance on estrus and the old culture, in other words, voluntary action. L. S. Vygotsky,[3] the prominent psychologist, felt that it is reasonable to think that our voluntary actions, more than our advanced intellect, distinguishes humans from our closest animal relatives.

Interestingly, with regard to the chimpanzee, who is our closest animal relative, evolutionary biologists, Johan Lind and Patrik Lindenfore, of the University of Stockholm, using previously collected data about chimpanzee communities, came to the conclusion that female chimpanzees are the carriers of culture.[4] The authors state that female chimpanzees express and transmit more culture than male chimpanzees. They found that the number of cultural traits present in a chimpanzee community correlates with the average number of females in the community but not with the average number of males. Exactly what bearing this has on our human situation is not known, but it is of interest because this book gives much credit to females for human culture, and we see that female importance to chimpanzee culture may be a precedent for this.

Since sexual breast love is cultural, there are women who do not indulge in it, but there is reason to believe that at one time it was a universal, or nearly universal, human practice. Today, despite the negative effects of technology on transmission of the practice, it is likely the basis of many successful relationships. Unfortunately, as Donald S. Marshall commented, the use of the breast during sex may be a practice of the cognoscenti – implying a general lack of education on this topic.[5]

Sexual breast love may have been only an occasional experience at first, before it was culturally embraced on a universal or nearly universal basis. Perhaps its cultural adoption occurred under difficult circumstances, involving a struggle for survival. This is one of the imponderables in human development. Under ordinary circumstances it might have been difficult or impossible for an early human community to accept this method of relating, going against the natural sexuality of estrus and the prevailing early human culture of male sexual dominance. According to neuroscientist Antonio Damasio, human freedom may seem to be restricted by biology and culture, but people do have some opportunity for "willing and performing actions that may go against the apparent grain of biology and culture" to achieve "a new level of being." [6]

The adult erotic use of the breast before and during copulation changed sexual intercourse from an obligatory event, controlled to a large extent by nature and involving some unknown amount of physical pleasure, to an act of self-directed desire and well defined pleasure. The breast became an organ of culture. William Calvin points out that in evolution there is a great deal of multiple use of body structures.[7] According to him, the original function of an organ does not have to disappear. In the case of the breast, the feeding of offspring remains a basic mammary function. Although often not done by contemporary women, not long ago breast feeding provided the main nourishment given to an infant and was highly instrumental in establishing the maternal-infant bond. With the cultural spread of breast sex and the resultant bonding between men and women, the use of the breast was enhanced beyond its original function to include the forging of strong psychological bonds between the sexes. Both purposes remain important to the health of our species.

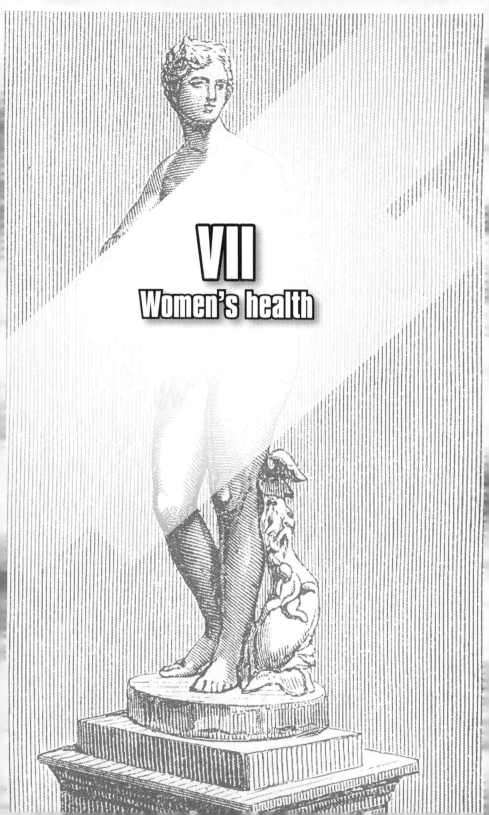

VII
Women's health

1

Sexual dysfunction, depression, and cancer

RESEARCH ON WOMEN'S HEALTH has shown that women exhibit certain unwanted conditions more than men. E. O. Laumann in the *The Journal of the American Medical Association (JAMA)*, for instance, reported in 1999 that sexual dysfunction in the U.S. was more prevalent in women than in men, with 43 percent of women affected, and 31 percent of men.[1] They stated that the occurrence of sexual dysfunction was more likely among those with poor emotional and physical well-being, and is associated to a high degree with negative experiences in sexual relationships and in over-all health. In unhappy marriages, women are three times more likely than men to be depressed, as found by McGrath in 1990;[2] and according to the American Psychological Association in 1996, women are approximately two times as likely than men to suffer from major depression.[3] Revealingly, in the 2010 National Survey of Sexual Health and Behavior, a large representative study of sexual behavior in the U.S. by Indiana University, only 64 percent of women said they had experienced orgasm the last time they had sex, as compared to men, most of whom said they had achieved orgasm, and 80 percent of whom believed their partner had also.[4]

Gynecological cancer, including cancers of the cervix, uterus, ovary, vagina, and vulva affected almost 90,000 women in the U.S. in 2012, the last two cancers being relatively rare, according to the National Cancer Institute. [5] The incidence of gynecological cancers in recent years has been somewhat reduced in the U.S., but the burden of gynecological cancers in other parts of the world is greater than in the U.S. Interestingly, breastfeeding has been implicated in risk reduction for in-situ cervical cancer,[6] endometrial cancer of the uterus,[7] and ovarian cancer.[8]

Breast cancer is the most common type of cancer in women. Susan G. Komen reports that in 2015 it was estimated that in the U.S. there would be approximately 232, 000 new cases of invasive breast cancer and 60,000 new cases of non-invasive breast cancer.[9] There would be 40,000 deaths from breast cancer. The number of women in the U.S. diagnosed with breast cancer today indicates a major epidemic, although the incidence of new breast cancer cases has been relatively stable for the last ten years.[10] Some attention has been paid to how to prevent breast cancer. For instance it has been shown by Valerie Beral and her research group that longer length of breast feeding is a factor in reducing the risk of breast cancer. [11]

Cultural and behavioral changes to functional breast use were emphasized in the etiology of breast cancer by the physician, Dr. Timothy. G. C. Murrell, a community health expert in Australia until his death in 2002.[12] He acknowledged the length of breast feeding as one such factor. In discussing the proper physiological functioning of the breasts, he suggested that sexual breast stimulation may be a variable in effecting a reduced risk of breast cancer, and that the amount of nipple erection over time might be a critical factor.

2

To find a cure, look within

THE BREASTS NOT ONLY feed the newborn and toddler, but, stimulated during coitus, induce the uterus to contract in sexual climax. The uterus not only bears and nurtures the fetus, it beats rhythmically with orgasm. Fear and ignorance of women's sexuality prevents us from recognizing that women's nurturing organs and child bearing organs are also our sexual organs. To do so seems somehow to violate the innocence of babies and children. Rather than participate in a re-evaluation of women's sexuality and its relationship to reproductive health, the medical profession appears to concentrate on cures, to the exclusion of prevention. The field of basic biological science also neglects the area of sex research. In our present cultural environment, the female breast and uterus are at risk. Witness the ongoing epidemic of breast cancer and the threat to the sexual wholeness of so many women by excessive hysterectomies. The breasts and uterus are still not regarded as the vital sexual organs that they are, and because of this misconception these organs are the sites of major and costly disease.

For women born today, one out of eight in the U.S. will be diagnosed with breast cancer in her lifetime, with little attention paid to how to prevent it – a situation that strikes fear into women's hearts. In the 1970's this figure had been one in ten, indicating a worsened situation from that time, not so long ago.[1] For much of the latter part of their adult lives, women are resigned to undergoing repeated mammogram tests to check for suspicious breast tissue. Mammography can aid in reducing the number of breast cancer deaths in women ages 40 to 70, but even with improved techniques, as many as twenty percent of cancers are missed; furthermore, false positives can occur, that is, diagnoses of abnormality when no cancer is present.[2] This causes anxiety and additional costly testing. There are also certain cancers that will never cause symptoms or need treatment, resulting in over-diagnosis by mammography, especially in women over age sixty-nine.

Once incurred, the management of breast cancer commands many resources. Of all medical costs associated with cancer in 2010, the highest cost, $16.5 billion was for breast cancer.[3] There are always new medicines in development for breast cancer, as well as drugs being developed to help patients deal with nausea and other side effects. This kind of research is fueled by the many cases of invasive breast cancer in women. However, according to the American Cancer Society, a sharp decrease of almost 7 percent in the breast cancer incidence rate between 2002 and 2003 can be attributed to a reduction in the use of menopausal hormone therapy, leaving an incidence rate that is now considered to be fairly steady.[4]

The idea of "the cure" for breast cancer, as publicized by the Susan G. Komen for the Cure Foundation is meant to be reassuring. Ironically, scientists tell us that they don't know what causes breast cancer, and they don't have a cure. But there have been some advances. According to the American Cancer Society, 90 out of 100 women who have breast cancer will survive for at least 5 years.[5] That's a 90 percent 5 year survival rate. If the cancer is caught early and confined to the breasts, the 5 year survival rate is 99 percent.

A combination of factors, including genes and lifestyle are posited in the development of cancer. Genetic causes are suspected when there is a family history of breast cancer, which is the case for 5 percent of patients. For other patients, lifestyle, which can be changed, and some unalterable factors are cited. Age is a very large risk factor, because 95 percent of all breast cancers occur in women over age 40. On the American Cancer Society website, among the lifestyle risk indicators are: being overweight, inactivity, daily alcohol consumption, long term use of menopausal hormone therapy, and not breastfeeding. A big question for women is: "What am I doing, or not doing, in my life that might cause breast cancer?" The lifestyle indicators provide some of the answers. Of particular interest has been the addition of "not breastfeeding" to the list of risk factors.

"To find a cure for breast cancer the first place you must look is within" was the advice of an advertisement by The Susan G. Komen Breast Cancer Foundation in a supplement to the *New York Times Magazine* in 1999.[6] This enigmatic advice undoubtably refers to the ritual of taking yearly diagnostic mammograms. But another way to look within would be to re-examine the way women's bodies have worked throughout the thousands of years of human culture, and to begin once again to use the breasts as they were used in the past – as both sexual and nutritive organs. Pertinent to this book's message is that, because of underlying biological factors, the "non- sexual breast" may be found to carry a breast cancer risk similar to that of the "non-breastfeeding breast." Such a finding would take research.

3

Breastfeeding

SINCE THE LATE 1970's breast feeding has had a limited resurgence in the United States. Promotion of breast feeding has come from various women's health groups and community sources, with medical professionals at first officially endorsing it as a benefit to babies, but more recently as a benefit to women in lowering the risk of breast cancer. Rates of breast feeding initiation after birth have tripled in the last few decades. In 2010, 77 percent of mothers nursed their newborns, as compared to 24 percent in 1971, a sign of progress, but there is concern that babies are not breastfed for as long as recommended. The Center for Disease Control and Prevention (CDC) publishes breastfeeding data from the National Immunization Survey which is used here.[1] Of infants born in 2010, 49 percent were breastfed at 6 months, up from 35 percent in 2000. The breastfeeding rate at 12 months increased from 16 percent to 27 percent over the same period. One way to read these statistics is that women are willing to listen to recommendations and begin breastfeeding, but do not enjoy it over the long-term. A look at the backgrounds of women who breastfeed and those who do not, suggests a different story, one of social factors such as income, education, tradition, and work conditions.

A demographic profile of women who breastfeed their infants in the United States is available from Ross Laboratories Women's Survey.[2] In 2000, the initiation of breastfeeding was among the highest for mothers who were white, college educated, 35 or more years of age, and employed part-time; they were typically not enrolled in the Women, Infants, and Children (WIC) program for low income families, and they lived in the western U.S. and New England. This summary from Ross Laboratories provides information which they use to market formula. High rates of initial breastfeeding were found among Asian women and Hispanic women, whose cultures support breastfeeding. The women with the highest rates of breastfeeding their six and twelve months-old infants were essentially this same group. Women of Hispanic origin showed the influence of former life ways. Studies done in Mexico point out that Hispanic women have traditionally breastfed their babies throughout the past century, although the practice is now diminishing.

Mothers who were not employed outside the home were more likely to breastfeed their six and twelve-month-olds than women who were employed full or part time. Rates of breastfeeding initiation in the hospital were lowest among women who were African-American, grade school educated, less than 20 years of age, and employed full time; they were often participants in the WIC program for low income families, and lived in the southeast and central regions of the U.S.

It is especially distressing that women enrolled in the Women, Infant, and Children program, a public health initiative of the U.S. government, do not have a higher rate of breastfeeding, although the ultimate decision to nurse must always be a personal one. Adequate nutrition is clearly a public health issue for infants in poor areas where infant mortality rates are often very high, sometimes double the national average. Human breast milk provides the best infant nutrition, and women would benefit from intense education on this topic. Of equal importance, and it can't be stressed enough, is that, for the mother, breastfeeding her children reduces her risk of breast cancer, one of the top public health problems currently faced by women in the United States.

Unfortunately, a large barrier to poor women's ability to breastfeed was erected when the U.S. government decided to limit welfare assistance in 1996. The low wage jobs that most poor women must take provide neither the time nor the facilities to enable women to breastfeed their infants or to use the breast pump to reserve their milk for later bottle use. There is also the issue of good nutrition for the nursing mother, and the fact that poor women may not have the income nor even the food-stamps to obtain nutritious food for themselves is an obstacle to breastfeeding.

What is clear from the foregoing profile is that for most women, long term breastfeeding is a luxury. The modern setting makes breastfeeding difficult for a variety of reasons including work constraints and the low valuation placed on it by society. Even with official recommendations, there is little social support for it unless a woman is middle class, educated, and can afford to stay at home. The exceptions are for those women with ethnic families who approve and help out. Alternative infant foods are readily available, making breastfeeding appear unnecessary and extravagant to some, and even strange and indecent to others.

There is a great deal of cultural uneasiness in the United States about a mother nursing a toddler, and women who breastfeed beyond early infancy may face criticism, and sometimes, charges of child abuse. For instance, in 2000, a social service agency removed a five year old child from his home because his mother was still breastfeeding him.[3] The judge said that the extended breastfeeding created a situation with a large potential for emotional damage. The mother claimed that she intended to wean the child when he asked to stop breastfeeding, a practice supported by the American Academy of Pediatrics. The Academy recommended in 1997 that breastfeeding continue for at least 12 months, and after that for as long as mutually desired.[4]

How do women feel about their experiences of breastfeeding for more than an initial period after giving birth? To answer this question we turn to a locale where long-term breast feeding has been a traditional practice. Women from the Ugandan countryside were asked this question by developmental psychologist Mary D. Ainsworth.[5] The women indicated whether or not they enjoyed nursing their babies. Three women in the study said that they felt a special pleasure when they breast-fed their babies. One young woman admitted that she liked breast feeding so much that she was hesitant to wean her child although he was walking and over a year old. Ainsworth says that fourteen mothers indicated unreservedly that they enjoyed breastfeeding. Two others tempered their endorsement, one saying that she liked the idea of nursing someone she felt affection for, and the other that she liked it because it was good for her child. Six women said that they had enjoyed breastfeeding at first, but that it had become troublesome after some months; four said they did not enjoy it at all. There are mixed feelings about breastfeeding, even in this rural setting in the non-Western world, a place where mothers more typically do it for longer periods.

Women may find the experience enjoyable, but also challenging. A potential hurdle to long-term breastfeeding is the demand it presents on the body's resources. Breastfeeding involves the senses and elicits pleasurable sensations, but at the same time it is physically demanding, especially when continued for many months. At first, extra energy is not needed to produce the milk, but after the first six weeks, if no infant formula supplement is used, the process of breastfeeding burns 500 to 600 calories a day. Without good nutrition, the mother may begin to feel fatigued. The addition of soft solid foods to the baby's diet starting at about six months may create a small dent in the work of making breast milk, but not if the rate of nursing remains the same. Adding cow's milk or soy milk, and gradual weaning, ideally not before one year, allows breastfeeding to linger on at a less demanding level for as long as mother and child desire-- a laudable outcome.

Breastfeeding is an experience of bodily sensations and secretions. The initial let-down or arrival of the milk may be accompanied by pressure or a slight ache in the breasts. Many women must reduce distractions to a minimum and center their thoughts on the baby – allowing the milk to flow. In the best of circumstances, the baby easily latches onto the nipple and areola, and sucking begins, creating a fulfilling experience for both mother and baby. The mutual feeling of love that breastfeeding can bring is described in a study from Kenya by anthropologist Robert Alan LeVine in which a baby's enthusiasm for nursing and a mother's happiness in indulging her child make clear the reciprocal relationship.[6] The baby drinks from the plenty of the breasts, relieving the mother, while the mother's milk satisfies the baby. Mother and baby together establish a mutual loving relationship with its own distinct perceptions and enjoyments.

4

Women build a movement

BREAST CANCER IS SOMETIMES described as a mysterious illness, a designation that does not inspire confidence that it can be cured. But we do have time in our daily lives to try to prevent the disease. A clear strategy would be for more women to breastfeed their babies beyond six months for at least a year, as recommended by the American Academy of Pediatrics.[1] Whereas in 1978 the Academy cited the nutritional advantage of breastfeeding to babies, since 1997 they have also cited the advantage to women in lessening the risk of breast cancer.

Even before the 1978 pediatric recommendation, women's initiative had created a movement toward better health – a phenomenon that started in the early 1960s when, without any clear directives from physicians, some women in industrialized countries began to return to the practice of breast feeding their infants. La Leche League International, founded in the U.S. by a few women in Chicago, quickly grew to a multinational effort that effectively questioned the rejection of functional breast use that had been current in the 1930s through the 1950s. These women criticized the use of formula in bottles for infant feeding and in 1963 they aided women to reach breastfeeding goals by publishing *The Womanly Art of Breastfeeding.*[2] Shortly afterwards, a related movement concerned with women's health and sexuality became prominent, an offshoot of the feminist movement of the time. Relatively well informed women made basic knowledge about women's bodies more widely available with the publication in 1973 of *Our Bodies, Ourselves,*[3] referred to by evangelical minister Jerry Falwell as "obscene trash."[4] These two books were part of the pioneering effort to make women more aware of their own health needs and those of their children.

Public awareness campaigns continue to emphasize the responsibility of formula manufacturers in infant disease around the world. These businesses, by their interference with breastfeeding, are also culpable in the growing incidence of breast cancer worldwide. The breastfeeding movement remains active today, not only promoting infant nutrition, but serving as a kind of self-help anti-cancer movement.

Receiving support and good advice is one thing, but implementing it is quite another, especially when a woman must work. Women may like the idea of breastfeeding, but to carry it out in the long term is challenging. Balancing work, baby, and a complex of other chores and commitments requires resourcefulness on the part of a nursing mother. Gale Pryor in her book *Nursing Mother, Working Mother* elucidates the many difficulties that women face on the job.[5] She notes that breastfeeding often means carrying the baby everywhere, but that for most working women, keeping the baby close by is not an option. Pumping breast milk for bottle use is one solution when jobs take women away from home. According to Pryor, new equipment on the market makes the process possible, but pumping at work raises other problems. For instance, sustained closeness to the infant is often essential to bring in an adequate milk supply, and frequency of feeding is preferable, otherwise the supply begins to dwindle. These daunting practical aspects of long term breastfeeding make it apparent that for many women breastfeeding is just not possible.

5

Prevention

THE LONGER WOMEN BREASTFEED their babies, the more they are protected against breast cancer. So says an important study from England on lactation and cancer published by Valerie Beral and her group in the *Lancet* in the summer of 2002.[1] This conclusion was reached after collecting and reanalyzing research done throughout the world on breastfeeding. Longer duration of breastfeeding, if carried out to a greater extent in developed countries would have social, medical, and economic benefits.

But the authors of the *Lancet* article were somewhat pessimistic in outlook. Although they encouraged women to lengthen the period of breastfeeding, they predicted that a return to a lifestyle abandoned almost a century ago might not be realistic for many women. They put their hope instead in finding the mechanism by which breastfeeding provides protection. They felt that it might be possible to mimic the effects of breastfeeding therapeutically.

One prospect is that the effects of breastfeeding can be mimicked by the sexual use of the breasts. It is already known that breastfeeding and sexual breast use are related, both involving an increase in oxytocin, though for the non-lactating breast this increase has so far been shown to be limited to one part of the menstrual cycle. There are no statistics on the number of women who use their breasts sexually, and little or no information at all delving deeper into the subject. For instance, it would be interesting to know if milk is produced in small amounts with sexual breast use. Related to this, it has been shown that for adoptive mothers who attempt to breastfeed, nipple stimulation induces a small amount of lactation.[2] Further research in this area would provide a needed advance in the science of women's health.

In Mexico, studies of long term lactation are facilitated by a public health sector that promotes nursing.[3] Prolonged breastfeeding has been a way of life in Mexico until recently, and researchers there saw some protective effect after as little as three months of lactation and the effect was major after three or more years. Extended nursing has been widespread in China,[4] and also in Japan,[5] where research has shown similar protective results. In Hong Kong, women from fishing villages practice an unusual traditional kind of nursing. The women of the Chinese Tanka, or boat people, construct their clothing with the front opening always on the right side, a design which makes it convenient to use exclusively the right breast in nursing. Investigation of cancer development in postmenopausal women there revealed a highly significant increase of cancer risk in the unused breast.[6]

In a somewhat analogous model with lactating mice, researchers experimentally prevented access to the nipple on one side, and the mice were exposed to chemicals.[7] More tumors were produced on the blocked side because breast tissues there endured prolonged exposure to carcinogen. On the suckled side, the carcinogen was excreted in the milk and could not be metabolically activated by breast tissue.

How does prolonged breastfeeding work to protect against breast cancer? Scientists have proposed several pathways.
1. Physical changes in breast tissue accompany milk production or lactation which causes some cells of the breast

to differentiate, that is, to mature in a healthy way. This differentiation potentially reduces the cells' susceptibility to carcinogenic processes.[8]

2. Transforming growth factor B is a substance found in the human body and it is secreted during lactation. TGF-B is a regulator of cell growth, and has been described as having high potential to inhibit the growth of human breast cancer cells.[9]

3. Harmful concentrations in the breast of potential carcinogens are reduced by lactation. These include toxic chemicals such as DDT and other environmental contaminants. Oxytocin, which causes the breast cells to contract, is a factor in the elimination of these chemicals.[10]

4. During lactation a woman's ovulation cycles and menstruation are suppressed when the baby is totally breast fed. When she is not ovulating, a woman's estrogen levels are lower, which could inhibit initiation or growth of breast cancer.[11] Once supplementary feeding is started, ovulation and menstruation usually return.

Despite accumulating evidence that lactation reduces the risk of breast cancer, most scientists and doctors, until recently, thought it premature to advise women to breastfeed as an aid to their own health. The American Academy of Pediatrics was the exception, and in their 1997 directive, they listed the following possible health benefits for women who breastfeed: the reduced risk of premenopausal breast cancer, the reduced risk of ovarian cancer, and the increased levels of oxytocin that cause diminished bleeding after childbirth. To be expected, they stressed the incomparable value of breast milk for infants. Their policy statement advised: "Extensive research, especially in recent years, documents diverse and compelling advantages to infants, mothers, families, and society from breastfeeding."[12]

The authors of the 2002 *Lancet* study, above, concluded that: If women in developed counties have, on the average, 2.5 children, and breastfeed each child for six months longer than they currently do, about 25,000 breast cancers (5 percent) could be prevented each year. They projected that 50,000 breast cancers (11 percent) might be prevented if women breastfed each child for twelve months more than they do at present. It is clear that impressive health benefits would accrue to women by making it possible for them to follow this advice.

Without significant societal change, it's difficult to imagine that breastfeeding lasting for a year or more will again become prevalent in the West. Wide cultural adoption of breastfeeding would require a more equitable world with large-scale interventions on behalf of public health. Some solutions might be: a paid six-month maternity leave from the work place; hospital practices designed to overcome the difficulties of breastfeeding at the start; and while at home, support from public health clinics. On the level of a complete economic transformation, a shorter work week with no reduction in income would allow both parents to spend more time with their children and facilitate breastfeeding and other healthy practices. This solution would offer a substantial boost to the health of the planet.

6

Science, education, and the sexual breast

SCIENCE HAS NOT EXPENDED much time thinking about the relationship between sex and health, resulting in an area that is moribund. Although science has recognized a health benefit with breastfeeding, the exact mechanism of nursing's effect in reducing the risk of breast cancer has yet to be determined. The baby, while feeding, innocently caresses and sucks its mother's breast and reduces her risk of cancer. Hypotheses as to how this is accomplished suggest various biological processes as outlined in the last section, but more research is needed, extending as well to the sexual breast.

Because of similarities to breastfeeding, breast sex or nipple eroticism, may also reduce the risk of cancer by a parallel mechanism. Research in this area would be crucial to women's self knowledge. Although there are other ways to facilitate sexual climax, for instance with the clitoris, the sexual use of the breast may be the healthiest way to aid in reaching orgasm. Furthermore, while breastfeeding takes place in a well defined and more or less limited time span, breast sex involves the functional use of the breasts over a lifetime, suggesting a promising long term health strategy and lifestyle.

An investigation done in Japan in the 1950's is compelling, as reported by Quisenberry: after interviewing women with breast cancer as well as those without it about their lives, the researcher, Dr. T. Hariyama, found that "caressing of the breast" apparently protects against breast cancer.[1] Caressing the breast is a technique of breast sex or sexual breast love, defining a particular sexual lifestyle, and Dr. Hariyama's findings indicate a good reason to use a lifestyle approach in the study of sexual health and disease. Because of the epidemic nature of breast cancer, many research strategies for investigating the causes of breast cancer are desirable, including holistic lifestyle studies.

Dr. Hariyama determined that breast cancer in Japan seemed to be more prevalent in women who had adopted a Western style of living. This information was cited in Quisenberry's article about socio-cultural factors related to cancer in Hawaii. The article stated that for Japanese women living in Hawaii, cancer of the breast appeared to be increasing. Change in these women's love-making habits to conform to a more Caucasian pattern was named as a possible reason for the increase. Caucasian life style can be equated with modern living in a complex technological world, where despite the supposed sexual freedom of young adults and the quantity of published material on sexual techniques, many lose touch with their sexuality.

Teen health and its relationship to teen sexual practice is the start of a lifelong story of sex and its influence on well-being. According to the Kinsey Institute, the average age of first intercourse in the United States is 16.9 years for males and 17.4 years for females.[2] The sexual use of the breast by teen age women merits elucidation, but studies of teen sexuality tend to focus on the vulnerability of teens to high risk sexual practices, as well as on the incidence of pregnancy, contraceptive use, and sexually transmitted disease.

A Canadian study of sexual health by Hanson, Mann, McMahon, and Wong observes that there is a reluctance by survey takers and health researchers to directly question younger people about various sexual issues.[3] The authors felt that, in order to fairly measure sexual health, researchers must use a broad definition of sexuality. This reluctance to question frankly, and a narrow understanding of sex, might explain the paucity of information about sexual breast use. The National Survey of Sexual Health and Behavior of 2010, conducted by Indiana University, with 5,865 respondents ages 14 to 94, including about 800 under the age of 18, did take a broader look at sexuality, and found that the sexual practices of teens are as varied as those of adults, but the study did not specifically document the incidence of sexual breast use.[4]

A study of particular interest was conducted in 2006 by Levin and Meston concerning nipple/breast stimulation during the sexual activity of young people.[5] They administered a short questionnaire to sexually experienced undergraduates between 17 and 29 years of age, with 95 percent between ages 18 and 22. With regard to the women, numbering 153, about 82 percent reported that stimulation of their nipples/breasts caused or enhanced their sexual arousal; 78 percent agreed that when already aroused, such manipulation increased their arousal; and 59 percent said that they had asked to have their nipples stimulated during lovemaking. Of the men, 148 in number, 52 percent reported that such stimulation caused or enhanced their sexual arousal. From the standpoint of the present discussion, these respondents can be considered the cognoscenti of young people.

Susanna Schrobsdorff writes in *Time* magazine about the current generation of adolescents between the ages of 12 and 18 years in the U.S.[6] She notes research showing that teenage girls are far more likely to experience depression than teenage boys. About 20 percent of girls and 6 percent of boys totaling 3 million teens had a major depressive episode in 2015. These numbers had recently gone up, and represent 12.5 percent of the teen population of that year. Girls also outnumbered boys in experiencing anxiety, 30 percent girls to 20 percent boys, adding up to 6.3 million teens or 25 percent of the teen population. Self harm such as self-cutting is an activity accompanying depression in some of today's teens: 60 percent to 70 percent of those who have ever self-injured are girls. Blood and pain make these teens feel more real and connected to the body, according to researchers, suggesting a sexual problem at base, but the article places the blame largely on cell phone culture and related stress.

Concerning a fundamental cultural practice such as breast sex, education is a necessity, especially in advanced industrial society among youth. There are no longer village elders and large extended families who instruct in such matters, although in close ethnic communities this information is sometimes passed down from mother to daughter or shared among good friends. In other situations teens must rely on sex education in the schools for an understanding of their bodies.

According to an article by Landry, Singh, and Darroch concerning sex education in the fifth and sixth grades in the United States, beginning in these grades and continuing over the next few years, the changes of puberty are expected to be taught in many public schools.[7] This includes instruction on the functions of organs, glands, and hormones, and their effects on sexual behavior, feelings, and general behavior. Information about the sexuality of the breast and uterus would easily fit into such a program. However there are many difficulties attendant on sex education, and the authors of this article conclude that schools are doing little to prepare students for puberty and future sexual activity. One might add that the general health as well as the sexual health of young people may be improved by sex education.

Returning again to Dr. Timothy Murrell of Adelaide University, his idea for a long term health approach to preventing breast cancer included the ongoing elimination of carcinogens that collect in the glands of the breasts.[8] He suggested that the practice of nipple care, as he termed it, whether in conjunction with a partner during sex, or through self-care, might have the capacity to eliminate mammary carcinogens. Three categories of oxytocin production – with sex, with self nipple care, and with breastfeeding – were felt by Murrell to be important. This theory of breast cancer prevention is based on the increase in oxytocin that comes about with nipple stimulation and the concomitant contraction of the myoepithelial cells of the breast and possible expulsion of carcinogens. However, future research on oxytocin release with nipple stimulation is necessary to understand women's sexuality and breast cancer, as discussed by Murrell.

In addition to its theorized role in breast cancer prevention, oxytocin secreted into the body with suckling at the breast has a role in maintaining the health of the uterus, and is utilized in obstetrics today. Oxytocin is a first line treatment for postpartum hemorrhage. Oxytocin stimulates the uterus to contract rhythmically, which constricts spiral arteries and decreases blood flow through the uterus.[9] In addition, it is well known that putting the baby to suckle at the breast immediately after childbirth helps to stop the sometimes excessive bleeding that follows delivery. In this regard, Chua in 1994 showed that when an infant begins to nurse right after its birth there is an increase of uterine activity of ninety-three percent on the average.[10]

In traditional medical practice dating back thousands of years, mechanical suction of the breasts known as "cupping" was used to ease heavy menstrual flow. Helen King in her study of the female body in ancient Greece notes that both Hippocrates and Soranus advocated this method to relieve women's menstrual distress.[11] These early physicians treated both heavy periods and postpartum bleeding in this way. The "cup" is a device still used in traditional medicine today as a means to generate uterine contractions, as advertised on the internet. In the past, the cups were warmed and placed on the nipples, and as they cooled, they produced suction. Today, suction machines are available on the internet from China for this purpose.

Prompted by this traditional remedy, it would be instructive to research the effect of the sexual use of the breasts in the quelling of heavy periods. Consider the alternative: more than one third of the approximately 700,000 hysterectomies performed each year in the United States are for excessive uterine bleeding, with one third to one half of these showing no structural abnormality, according to Cooper and Erickson.[12] Hysterectomy in these latter cases appears to be an extreme remedy for a condition that is a variant of normal.

The possible efficacy of breast sex in maintaining uterine health is suggested by a study by Brock that shows that a reduced risk for in-situ cervical cancer occurs with a history of breastfeeding.[13] This adds points to an impressive health score for breastfeeding as a protection against diseases of the reproductive tract. Breastfeeding has been implicated in risk reduction not only for in-situ cervical cancer, but also for endometrial cancer of the uterus as shown by Newcomb,[14] and for ovarian cancer as determined by Grimes.[15] Although the exact mechanism of the protective effect of breastfeeding in these cases has not been worked out, the increased uterine activity associated with nursing, as also found with the sexual use of the breasts, comes to mind as a possible factor. An integrative approach to women's reproductive health is worth examining. Functional use of the breasts in lovemaking provides just such a comprehensive experience, engaging both uterus and breasts in an agenda for healthier sex organs.

Conclusion

OUR CONTEMPORARY CULTURE AND woman's second class status in it undermines women's sexual and general health. This book invokes the earliest of modern human epochs and the idea that women were not always subordinate participants in society, but rather the earliest shapers of human culture. It is contended that breast sex was the first characteristic cultural practice of modern humankind. The act of breast sex cannot rely on instinct, and, in the absence of permissive and fortuitous experimentation, it requires learning. Culture depends on learning and the transmission of ideas to successive generations, and the culture of women's sexuality is not immune from these requirements. Women's isolation from the decision making centers of society allows her needs to be neglected, even belittled, including her sexual health needs, an issue of great concern here.

Scientific investigation is crucial to confirm that the uterus and breasts are sexual organs, and that breast sex is a practice basic to women's health. Citing current information on oxytocin, a hormone and neurotransmitter of the human body, this book has tried to show how the breasts and uterus are integrated in their sexual function, and how women's sex lives can blossom with this realization. It is hoped that this account will encourage research and education pertaining to human female sexuality. Further understanding of this area will undoubtedly confer important healthful benefits on women, notably amelioration of sexual dysfunction, reduction in the number of unnecessary hysterectomies, and perhaps, even prevention of breast cancer.

The uses of the breast, to love and feed the infant and to promote the emotional tie between female and male, have been fundamental to the human way of life. Despite breastfeeding's continued value in nourishing the child, and its efficacy in mother and child bonding, breastfeeding as the major source of infant food is disappearing in the developed world. This happens even though there is evidence to show that breastfeeding has a role in cancer prevention in the mother and is very beneficial to the infant. The sexual use of the breast may also be disappearing in Western type societies, but unfortunately there is no information on this subject. There is little education or knowledge concerning this formerly vital practice – with perhaps critical consequences for women and humanity.

The human art of teaching, which propagates human culture and sociality from generation to generation, has been suppressed, or at least the teaching of love and sharing that could keep our complex world from disintegrating. Our early ancestors probably depended mostly on observation and imitation to learn, but we are now highly dependent on complex instruction, a key to our behavior. Not of least importance, should be the teaching of cultural sexuality, which has been done in other societies, as documented in the ethnographic record. Ironically in the supposedly most advanced societies, for instance, in the United States, sex education is confronted with many obstacles.

In maintaining the health of our social existence, a culture of love depends on a relationship of equality between women and men. There is a constant tendency for dominance and aggression to be reasserted, negating love and allowing women and other large segments of society to be devalued. To the extent that this power and hostility are accepted and instated, oppression and repression occur, and of special concern here, the degradation of women. Domestic suffering caused by dysfunctional sexuality, and its consequence, dysfunctional family life, can be tied to the lack of appreciation of women's potential. Of particular importance, and the purpose of this text, is to acknowledge women's unique sexuality and its place at the nexus of biology and culture. A new understanding of women's sexuality is necessary. Women's practice of sexual breast love has implications not only for women's health but for the health of our world. Renewing a society based on functional sexuality and its attendant functional family life, is a step in keeping us from life-ways characterized mainly by dominance relations – for which there is strong evidence in today's world. The ancient project of establishing love and equality in human relations has yet to be realized in modern times, although we set the stage for it long ago with woman's initiation of cultural sexuality.

Notes/Reading

Introduction: A unique feminine way of sex
1. Timothy G. C. Murrell, "Epidemiological and Biochemical Support for a Theory on the Cause and Prevention of Breast Cancer," *Medical Hypotheses* 36 (1991): 389-396.
2. Timothy G. C. Murrell, "The Potential for Oxytocin (OT) to Prevent Breast Cancer: A Hypothesis," *Breast Cancer Research and Treatment* 35 (1995): 225-229.
3. Shere Hite, *The Hite Report: A Nationwide Study of Female Sexuality* (New York: Seven Stories Press, 2004).
4. Naomi Wolfe, *Vagina: A New Biography* (New York: HarperCollins Publishers, 2012).
5. V. C. Robinson, "Support For the Hypothesis That Sexual Breast Stimulation Is An Ancestral Practice and A Key tTo Understanding Women's Health," *Medical Hypotheses 85 (2015): 976-985.*
6. A. C. Kinsey and the Staff of the Institute for Sex Research, Indiana University. *Sexual Behavior of the Human Female* (Philadelphia: W. B.Saunders, 1953).
7. C. S. Ford & F. A. Beach, *Patterns of Sexual Behavior* (New York: Harper, 1951).

Chapter I: Cultural sexuality and the biology of love

1. The sexual breast

1. Marilyn Yalom, *A History of the Breast* (New York: Alfred A. Knopf, Inc, 1997).
2. Joyce Carol Oates, "Landfill," *The New Yorker,* October 9, 2006.
3. Haruki Murakami, "Town of cats," *The New Yorker,* September 5, 2011.
4. C.S. Ford and F.A. Beach, *Patterns of Sexual Behavior* (New York: Harper, 1951).
5. Paul H. Gebhard, "Human Sexual Behavior: A Summary Statement," in *Human Sexual Behavior: Variations in the Ethnographic Spectrum* ed. Donald S. Marshall and Robert C. Suggs (New York/London: Basic Books, Inc, 1971), 209.
6. Y. Yuge, in Japanese, "The Effect of Interdependency on Levels of Self and Other Perception," *Shinrigaku Kenkyo* 67(31) (Aug, 1996): 177-85.
7. Robert C. Suggs and Donald S. Marshall, "Anthropological Perspectives on Human Sexual Behavior," in *Human Sexual Behavior: Variations in the Ethnographic Spectrum,* ed. Donald S. Marshall and Robert C. Suggs (New York: Basic Books, Inc, 1971), 219.
8. W. H. Masters and V. E. Johnson, *The Human Sexual Response* (Boston: Little, Brown, 1966).

2. The family and the human pair-bond

1. George Peter Murdock, *Social Structure* (New York: Macmillan, 1949).
2. Nancy Makepeace Tanner, *On Becoming Human* (New York: Cambridge University Press, 1981).
3. Frederick Engels, *The Origin of the Family, Private Property, and the State* (New York: International Publishers, 1970), 5-6, 40, 43, 48, 58, 145.

4. Bernard Chapais, *Primeval Kinship: How Pair Bonding Gave Birth to Human Society* (Cambridge, MA: Harvard University Press, 2008).

5. Zoltan Kovecses, *Emotion Concepts* (New York: Springer-Verlag, 1990), 132.

6. Robert J. Sternberg, "A Triangular Theory of Love," *Psychological Review* 93, no.2 (2007): 119-135.

7. A. C. Kinsey and the Staff of the Institute for Sex Research, Indiana University, *Sexual Behavior of the Human Female* (Philadelphia: W. B. Saunders, 1953).

8. Desmond Morris, *The Naked Ape: A Zoologist's Study of the Human Animal* (New York, McGraw-Hill, 1967), 63, 78.

9. J. M. Gottman, R. Tyson, K.R. Swanson, C.C. Swanson, and J.D. Murray, *The Mathematics of Marriage: Dynamic Nonlinear Models* (Cambridge, Mass: The MIT Press, 2003).

10. Theodosius Dobzhansky, *Mankind Evolving: The Evolution of the Human Species* (New Haven and London: Yale University Press, 1971), 199.

3. The breast and the love hormone

1. Jane Goodall, *The Chimpanzees of Gombe* (Cambridge, Massachusetts: The Belknap Press of Harvard University Press, 1986).

2. Robin Fox, *The Red Lamp of Incest: An Enquiry into the Origins of Mind and Society* (Notre Dame, Indiana: University of Notre Dame Press, 1983), 164.

3. Alice Rossi, "A Biosocial Perspective On Parenting," *Daedalus* 106 (1977): 1-33.

4. A.R. Fuchs, F. Fuchs, P. Husslein, M.S. Soloff, and M.J. Fernstrom, "Oxytocin Receptors and Human Parturition: A Dual Role for Oxytocin in the Initiation of Labor," *Science* 215 (1982): 1396-8.

5. K.L. Maughan, S.W. Heim, and S.S. Galazka, "Preventing Postpartum Hemorrhage: Managing the Third stage of Labor," *American Family Physician* 73(6) (2006): 1025-8.

6. D.W. Irons, P. Sriskandabalan, and C.H. Bullough, "A Simple Alternative to Parenteral Oxytocics for the Third Stage of Labor," *Int J Gynaecol Obstet* 46(1) (1994):15-18.

7. A.S. McNeely, I.C. Robinson, M.J. Houston, and P.W. Howie, "Release of Oxytocin and Prolactin in Response to Suckling," *Br Med J (Clin Res Ed)* 286(6361) (1983):257-9

8. M.S. Carmichael, R. Humbert, J. Dixen, G. Palmisano, W. Greenleaf, and J.M. Davidson, "Plasma Oxytocin Increases in the Human Sexual Response," *J Clin Endocrinol Metab* 64 (1987): 27-31.

9. W. Blaicher, D. Gruber, C. Bieglmayer, A.M. Blaicher, W. Knogler, and J.C. Huber, "The Role of Oxytocin in Relation to Female Sexual Arousal," *Gynaecol Obstet Invest* 47 (1999): 125-126.

10. J.A. Amico, and B.E. Finley, "Breast Stimulation in Cycling Women, Pregnant Women and a Woman with Induced Lactation: Pattern of Release of Oxytocin, Prolactin and Luteinizing Hormone," *Clin Endocrin (Oxf)* 25(2) (*1986*): 97-100.

11. R.D. Leake, J.E. Buster, and D.A. Fisher, "The Oxytocin Secretory Response to Breast Stimulation in Women During the Menstrual Cycle," *American Journal of Obstetrics and Gynecology* 148(4) (1984): 457-60.

12. A. Salonia, R.E. Nappi, M. Pontillo, R. Daverio, A. Smeraldi, A. Briganti, F. Fabbri, G. Zanni, P. Rigatti, and F. Montorsi, "Menstrual Cycle-Related Changes in Plasma Oxytocin Are Relevant to Normal Sexual Function in Healthy Women," *Hormonal Behavior* 47 (2) (2005): 164-9.

13. K.G. Auerbach and J.L. Avery, "Induced lactation: A Study of Adoptive Nursing by 240 Women," *American Journal of Diseases In Children* 135 (4) (1981): 340-3.

14. I. D. Neumann, "Brain Oxytocin: A Key Regulator of Emotional and Social Behaviours in Both Females and Males," *Journal of Endocrinology* 20(6) (Jun, 2008): 858-65.

15. D.M.Witt and T.R. Insel, "A Selective Oxytocin Antagonist Attenuates Progesterone Facilitation of Female Sexual Behavior," *Endocrinology.* 128(6) (Jun, 1991): 3269-76.
16. K.M. Kendrick, F. Levy, and E.B. Keverne, "Importance of Vaginocervical Stimulation for the Formation of Maternal Bonding in Primaparous and Multiparous Parturient Ewes," *Physiol Behav* 50(1991): 595-600.
17. J. Panksepp, B. Knutson, and D. L. Pruitt, "Toward a Neuroscience of Emotion: The Epigenetic Foundations of Emotional Development," in *What Develops in Emotional Development?* ed. Michael F. Mascolo and Sharon Griffin (New York: Plenum Press, 1998), 53-84.

4. Breast eroticism and the uterine connection

1. W.H Masters and V.E. Johnson, *The Human Sexual Response* (Boston: Little, Brown, 1966).
2. Marcel Mauss, *Sociology and Psychology: Essays,* trans. Ben Brewster (London; Boston: Routledge and Kegan Paul, Ltd.1979), 104.
3. Jonathan H. Slavin, "The Innocence of Sexuality," *Psychoanalytic Quarterly* LXXI (2002): 51-79.
4. Rossi, Alice, "A Biosocial Perspective on Parenting," *Daedalus 106 (1977): 1-33.*

5. The change to the family and the sharing of love

1. Melford D. Spiro, *Culture and Human Nature* (introduction), ed. B. Kilborne and L.L.Langness (New Brunswick, NJ: Transaction Publishers 1994), 265.
2. L.L. Langness, *The Study of Culture: Third Revised Edition* (Novato, CA: Chandler & Sharp Publishers, Inc, 1994), 256.
3. Edvard A. Westermarck. *The History of Human Marriage, 5th Edition.* London: Macmillan, 1921.
4. Jonathan H. Slavin. "The Innocence of Sexuality," *Psychoanalytic Quarterly LXXI* (2002): 51-79, p. 67.
5. Jonathan H. Slavin. Ibid. p.63.

6. Raymond DeCoccola, *The Incredible Eskimo: Life Among the Barren Land Eskimo* (Surrey, BC and Blaine, WA: Hancock House, 1986).

7. Sally Price, *Co-wives and Calabashes* (Ann Arbor: University of Michigan Press, 1993).

6. Incest in past human society

1. Geoffrey Gorer and J. H. Hutton, *Himalayan Village: An Account of the Lepchas of Sikkim* (London: Michael Joseph, Ltd, 1938).

2. Anne Baring and Jules Cashford, *Myth of the Goddess: Evolution of an Image* (New York: Viking Arkana, Penguin Books, 1991) Figure 32, page 267. Isis suckling her son, Horus, as a youth; c. 30 BCE – CE 14. Outer wall of Temple of Hathor, Denderah.

3. Sigmund Freud, *Totem and Taboo,* trans. James Strachey (New York: W. W. Norton and Co, 1952).

4. Robin Fox, *Kinship and Marriage: An Anthropological Perspective* (New York, NY: Cambridge University Press, 1996), 63 and 71-75.

5. Jane Goodall, *The Chimpanzees of Gombe* (Cambridge, Massachusetts: The Belknap Press of Harvard University Press, 1986).

6. C.R. Carpenter, "Sexual Behavior of Free Ranging Rhesus Monkeys (Macaca *mulatta*): II. Periodicity of Estrus, Homosexual, Autoerotic, and Non-conformist Behavior," *Journal of Comparative Psychology* 33(1) (February,1942): 143-162.

7. Penny Petrone, ed., *Northern voices: Inuit writing in English.* (Toronto: University of Toronto Press, 1988), 12.

8. Anne Baring and Jules Cashford, *The Myth of the Goddess: Evolution of an Image* (New York: Viking Arkana, Penguin Books, 1991).

9. Ibid, p. 251.

10. Bronislaw Malinowski, *Sex and Repression in Savage Society* (New York: Horace Liveright, 1927), 250.

Chapter II: The breast and human sexual behavior

1. The journey of the breast

1. Shere Hite, *The Hite Report: a Nationwide Study of Female Sexuality* (New York: Seven Stories Press, 2004), 78, 220, 321-324.
2. Daphne Ayalah and Isaac J. Weinstock, *Breasts: Women Speak About Their Breasts and Their Lives* (New York: Summit Books, 1979), 70, 153, 165-168, 178, 212.
3. Robert C. Suggs and Donald S. Marshall, "Anthropological Perspectives on Human Sexual Behavior," in *Human Sexual Behavior: Variations in the Ethnographic Spectrum,* ed. Robert S. Marshall and Robert C. Suggs (New York: Basic Books, Inc, 1971), 219.
4. Bronislaw Malinowski, *Sex and Repression in Savage Society* (New York: Horace Liveright, 1927), 250.
5. YouTube, *Who Owns the Breast; Street Talk Naija.* Accessed October 16, 2017. www.youtube.com/watch?v=qlvqiQOZdWY
6. Shere Hite, *The Hite Report*, 78.
7. Ibid., 220.
8. Ibid., 321-324.

2. The breast in the sex life of young people – sexual desire

1. Cora Alice DuBois, Abram Kardiner, and Emil Oberholzer, *The People of Alor: A Social-Psychological Study of an East Indian Island* (Minneapolis: Univ. of Minnesota Press, 1944), 98.
2. Bronislaw Malinowski, *Sex and Repression in Savage Society* (New York: Horace Liveright, 1927), 243, 250.

3. Robert Alan LeVine, *Gusii Sex Offences: A Study in Sexual Control* (Washington: American Anthropological Association, 1959), 975.

4. Charulal Mukherjea, *The Santals* (Calcutta: A. Mukherjee & Co., Private Ltd, 1962), 414.

5. Ibid., p. 414.

6. William George Archer, *The Hill of Flutes: Life, Love, and Poetry in Tribal India: Portrait of the Santals* (Pittsburgh: University of Pittsburgh Press, 1974), 124.

7. Ibid., p. 111.

8. Walter Dyk (Left Handed), *The Son of Old Man Hat: A Navaho Autobiography* (New York: Harcourt Brace and Company, 1938), 415.

9. Nils Magnus Holmer, *Cuna Chrestomathy* (Goteborg: Etnografiska Museet, 1951),157a.

10. Matthew Williams Stirling, *Historical and Ethnographical Material On the Jivaro Indians* (Washington: Govt. Print. Off, 1938), 109-110.

11. Donald Nathan Levine, *Wax &Gold: Tradition and Innovation in Ethiopian Culture* (Chicago: University of Chicago Press, 1965), 270.

3. Prohibitions against touching the breasts in courtship

1. Robert A. Orsi, *The Madonna of 115th Street: Faith and Community in Italian Harlem, 1880-1950* (New Haven, Connecticut: Yale University Press, 1958), 138.

2. Leopold J. Pospisil, *Kapauku Papuans and Their Law* (New Haven, Conn: Published for the Department of Anthropology, Yale University, 1958), 51.

3. Grenville Goodwin and Janice Thompson Goodwin, *The Social Organization of the Western Apache* (Chicago, Ill: The University of Chicago Press, 1942), 283.

4. Donald S. Marshall, *Cuna Folk: A Conceptual Scheme Involving the Dynamic Factors of Culture, As Applied to the*

Cuna Indians of Darien (New Haven: Human Relations Area Files, n.d.), 342.

4. The breasts in marriage and intercourse

1. Genevieve Calame-Griaule *Words and the Dogon World* (Philadelphia: Institute for the Study of Human Issues, 1986), 163.
2. Geza Roheim, *Women and Their Life in Central Australia* (London: The Institute, 1933), 240.
3. Charulal Mukherjea, *The Santals* (Calcutta: A. Mukherjee & Co., Private Ltd, 1962), 416.
4. William George Archer, *The Hill of Flutes: Life, Love, and Poetry in Tribal India: A Portrait of the Santals* (Pittsburgh: University of Pittsburgh Press, 1974), 98.
5. Thomas Gladwin and Seymour B. Sarason, *Truk: Man in Paradise* (New York: Wenner Gren Foundation for Anthropological Research, 1953), 110.
6. John L. Caughey, *Fa'a'nakkar Cultural Values in a Micronesian Society* (Philadelphia, Pa: Department of Anthropology, University of Pennsylvania, 1977), 114.
7. Donald S. Marshall, "Sexual Behavior on Mangaia". In D.S. Marshall and R.C. Suggs, eds, *Human Sexual Behavior* (New York: Basic Books, 1971), 114.
8. Ralph Linton, "Marquesan culture," in *The Individual and His Society: The Psychodynamics of Primitive Social Organization* by Abraham Kardiner, M.D. (New York: Columbia University Press, 1939), 173.
9. W.H. Masters and V.E. Johnson, *The Human Sexual Response* (Boston: Little, Brown, 1966).
10. Alice Rossi, "A Biosocial Perspective On Parenting," *Daedalus* 106 (1977): 1-33.
11. William R. Jankowiak, *Sex, Death, and Hierarchy in a Chinese City: An Anthropological Account* (New York: Columbia University Press, 1993), 234.

12. Gerardo Reichel-Dolmatoff and Sydney Muirden, *The Kogi: A Tribe of the Sierra Nevada de Santa Marta, Colombia. Vol. 2.* (Bogota: Editorial Iqueima, 1951), 286.

13. Gerardo Reichel-Dolmatoff and Sydney Muirden, *The Kogi: A Tribe of the Sierra Nevada de Santa Marta, Colombia. Vol. 1* (Bogota: El Instituto, 1949/1950), 273.

14. Robert Sutherland Rattray, *Ashanti Law and Constitution* (Oxford, England: Clarendon Press, 1929), 317.

15. Wayne Dennis, *The Hopi Child* (New York; D. Appleton-Century Company, Incorporated, for the Institute for Research in the Social Sciences, University of Virginia, 1940).

16. Thomas W. Maretzki, Hatsumi Maretski, and Beatrice B. Whiting, *Taira: An Okinawan Village* (New York: John Wiley and Sons, Inc, 1963), 430.

17. Cornelius Osgood, *The Koreans and Their Culture* (New York: The Ronald Press Company, 1951), 224.

18. Geoffrey Gorer and J. H. Hutton, *Himalayan Village: An Account of the Lepchas of Sikkim* (London: Michael Joseph, Ltd, 1938), 329.

19. George N. Appell, *The Nature of Social Groupings Among the Rungus Dusun of Sabah, Malaysia* (PhD Thesis. Australian National University, 1965), 55.

20. Havelock Ellis, *Studies In the Psychology of Sex. Volume I.* (Charleston SC: BiblioBazaar, 2006).

5. Denial of the sexual role of the breasts

1. Howard Keva Kaufman, *Bangkhuad: A Community Study in Thailand* (Locust Valley, N.Y.: Published for the Association for Asian Studies, 1960), 156.

2. Suzette Heald, *Controlling Anger: The Sociology of Gisu Violence* (Manchester, England: Manchester University Press, for the International African Institute, London, 1989), 218.

3. Tarunchandra Sinha, *The Psyche of the Garos* (Calcutta: Anthropological Survey of India, Govt. of India, 1966), 45.

4. M.C. Goswami and D.N. Majumdar, *A Study of Social Attitudes Among the Garo* (Calcutta: A. K. Bose, 1968), 57-58.

5. Lorna Marshall, *Marriage Among !Kung Bushmen* (London: Oxford University Press, 1959), 339.

6. Ronald Singer, *The Biology of the San* (Cape Town and Pretoria: Human & Rousseau, 1978), 122, 126.

7. Marjorie Shostak, *Nisa: The Life and Words of A !Kung Woman* (Cambridge, Mass: Harvard University Press, 1981), 166.

8. George B. Silberbauer, *Report to the Government of Bechuanaland On the Bushman Survey* (Gaberones: Bechuanaland Government, 1965).

9. Margaret Mead, *New Lives for Old: Cultural Transformation – Manus, 1928-1953* (New York: Morrow, 1956), 287.

10. Margaret Mead, *Kinship in the Admiralty Islands* (New York: American Museum of Natural History, 1934), 249.

11. Margaret Mead, *Growing Up In New Guinea: A Comparative Study of Primitive Education* (New York: W. Morrow & Company, 1930), 166.

12. Ibid., 59-61.

13. Reo Fortune, *Manus Religion: An Ethnological Study of the Manus Natives of the Admiralty Islands* (Philadelphia: The American Philosophical Society, 1935), 86-88.

Chapter III: Scenes from everyday life

1. Humor, sex, and the breast

1. Hugh Brooke Low and H. Ling Roth, "The Natives of Borneo: Edited From the Papers of the Late Brooke Low, Esq.," *Journal of the Anthropological Institute,* (August and November, 1892), 131.

2. Geoffrey Gorer and J. H. Hutton, *Himalayan Village: An Account of the Lepchas of Sikkim* (London: Michael Joseph, Ltd, 1938), 258.

3. John Morris, *Living With Lepchas: A Book About the Sikkim Himalayas* (London: William Heineman Ltd, 1938), 269.

4. Duncan Pryde. *Nunaga: My Land, My Country* (Edmonton, Alberta: M. G. Hurtig, Ltd, 1972), 82-83.

5. Andrei Simic, *Winners and Losers: Aging Yugoslavs in a Changing World* (Beverly Hills: Sage Publications, 1978), 89.

6. Willard Williams Hill, *Navaho Humor* (Menasha, Wis: George Banta Publishing Company, 1943).

2. The breast and joking among relatives

1. Margaret Mead, *Growing Up in New Guinea: A Comparative Study of Primitive Education* (New York: W. Morrow & Company, 1930), 59-61, 166. Margaret Mead, *Kinship in the Admiralty Islands* (New York: American Museum of Natural History, 1934) 249. Margaret Mead, *New Lives For Old: Cultural Transformation – Manus, 1928-1953* (New York: Morrow, 1956), 287.

2. Dennis O'Neil, "Marriage Rules: Part II Second Marriage Preferences." In *Sex and Marriage: An Introduction to the Cultural Rules Regulating Sexual Access and Marriage* anthro.palomar.edu. Accessed on November 12, 2015.

3. Max Gluckman, *Kinship and Marriage Among the Lozi of Northern Rhodesia and the Zulu of Natal* (London England: Oxford University Press, published for the International African Institute, 1958).

4. Sally Price, *Co-wives and Calabashes* (Ann Arbor: University of Michigan Press, 1993).

5. W.J. Culshaw, *Tribal Heritage: A Study of the Santals,* (London: Lutterworth Press, 1949).

6. Marine Carrin-Bouez and John Beierle, *Cultural Summary: Santal* (New Haven, Conn: Human Relations Area Files, 1998).

7. John G. Kennedy, *Tarahumara of the Sierra Madre: Beer, Ecology, and Social Organization* (Arlington Heights, Ill: AHM Pub. Corp, 1978).

8. Eugene A. Hammel, *Alternative Social Structures and Ritual Relations in the Balkans* (Englewood Cliffs, N. J.: Prentice-Hall, Inc., 1968).

3. Kinship and breast taboos

1. Roy Franklin Barton, *Ifugao Law* (Berkley: University of California Press, 1919).

2. John Roscoe, *The Bakitara or Bunyoro: The First Part of the Reprt of the Mackie Ethnological Expedition to Central Africa* (Cambridge, Eng.: The University Press, 1923).

3. Suzette Heald, *Controlling Anger: The Sociology of Gisu Violence* (Manchester, England: Manchester University Press, for the International African Institute, London, 1989).

4. Otto Friedrich Raum, *The Social Functions of Avoidances and Taboos Among the Zulu* (Berlin, New York: de Gruyter, 1973).

5. Thomas Gladwin and Seymour B. Sarason, *Truk: Man in Paradise* (New York: Wenner Gren Foundation for Anthropological Research, 1953), 110.

6. Dorothea Cross Leighton and Clyde Kluckhohn, *Children of the People: The Navaho Individual and His Development* (Cambridge: Harvard University Press, 1947).

7. William George Archer, *The Hill of Flutes: Life, Love, and Poetry in Tribal India: A Portrait of the Santals* (Pittsburgh: University of Pittsburgh Press, 1974).

8. Charulal Mukherjea, *The Santals* (Calcutta: A. Mukherjee & Co., Private Ltd., 1962), 415.

9. William George Archer, *The Hill of Flutes: Life, Love, and Poetry in Tribal India: A Portrait of the Santals* (Pittsburgh: University of Pittsburgh Press, 1974).

10. Charulal Mukherjea, *The Santals* (Calcutta: A. Mukherjee & Co., Private Ltd., 1962), 415.

4. Sex education from infancy to puberty and beyond

1. Sally Price, *Co-wives and Calabashes* (Ann Arbor: University of Michigan Press, 1993).
2. Raymond DeCoccola, *The Incredible Eskimo: Life Among the Barren Land Eskimo* (Surrey, BC and Blaine, WA: Hancock House, 1986).
3. Jean E. Jackson, *The Fish People: Linguistic Exogamy and Tukanoan Identity in Northwest Amazonia* (Cambridge and New York: Cambridge University Press, 1983).
4. Clyde Kluckhohn, *SomeAaspects of Navaho Infancy and Early Childhood* (New York, NY: International Universities Press, 1947).
5. William Howell, *The Sea Dyak* (New Haven: Human Relations Area Files, 1909).
6. Herbert Basedow, *The Australian Aboriginal* (Adelaide: F.W. Preece and Sons, 1925).
7. George Peter Murdock, "The Aranda of Central Australia," in *Our Primitive Contemporaries* (New York: The Macmillan Co, 1934) 20-47.
8. Geza Roheim, *The Eternal Ones of the Dream: A Psychoanalytic Interpretation of Australian Myth and Ritual* (New York: International Universities Press, 1945).
9. William George Archer, *Tribal Law and Justice: A Report on the Santal* (New Delhi: Concept, 1984).
10. John Morris, *Living with Lepchas: A Book About the Sikkim Himalayas* (London: William Heineman Ltd., 1938).

5. Breasts and the law

1. Leopold J. Pospisil, *Kapauku Papuans and Their Law* (New Haven, Conn.: Published for the Department of Anthropology, Yale University, 1958).
2. Robin Fox, *The Red Lamp of Incest: An Enquiry Into The Origins of Mind and Society* (Notre Dame, Indiana: University of Notre Dame Press, 1983), 164.

3. Hugh Brooke Low and H. Ling Roth, "The Natives of Borneo: Edited From the Papers of the Late Brooke Low, Esq." *Journal of the Anthropological Institute* (August and November, 1892), 131.

4. Laura W. R. Appell, *Menstruation Among the Rungus: An Unmarked Category* (Berkeley: University of California Press, 1988).

5. William George Archer, *The Hill of Flutes: Life, Love, and Poetry In Ttribal India: A Portrait of the Santals* (Pittsburgh: University of Pittsburgh Press, 1974).

6. Cora Alice DuBois, Abram Kardiner, and Emil Oberholzer, *The People of Alor: A Social-Psychological Study of an East Indian Island* (Minneapolis: Univ. of Minnesota Press, 1944).

7. Robert Sutherland Rattray, *Ashanti Law and Constitution* (Oxford, England: Clarendon Press, 1929).

8. Valentin A. Riasanovsky. *Fundamental Principles of Mongolian Law* (London: K. Paul, Trench, Tribner & Co., Ltd, 1937).

6. The breast at dances and ceremonies

1. Alcionilio Bruzzi Alves da Silva and Ivana Lillios, *The Indigenous Civilization of the Uaupes* (Sao Paulo: Centro de Pesquisas de Iauarete, 1962).

2. Geza Roheim, *Women and Their Life in Central Australia* (London: The Institute, 1933).

3. Simon David Messing, *The Highland Plateau Amhara of Ethiopia,* Lionel M. Bender, ed. 3 vols. (New Haven: HRAFlex Books, Human Relations Area Files, 1985).

4. William George Archer, *The Hill of Flutes: Life, Love, and Poetry in Tribal India: A Portrait of the Santals* (Pittsburgh: University of Pittsburgh Press, 1974).

5. Colin M.Turnbull, *The Forest People* (New York, NY: Simon and Schuster, 1962).

6. Irving Goldman, *The Cubeo: Indians of the Northwest Amazon* (Urbana, Illinois: University of Illinois Press, 1963).

7. Gerardo Reichel-Dolmatoff, *Amazonian Cosmos: The Sexual and Religious Symbolism of the Tukano Indians* (Chicago: the University of Chicago Press, 1971).

8. Grenville Goodwin and Janice Thompson Goodwin, *The Social Organization of the Western Apache* (Chicago, Ill: The University of Chicago Press, 1942).

9. Grenville Goodwin and Keith H. Basso, *The Western Apache Raiding and Warfare: From the Notes of Grenville Goodwin* (Tucson: University of Arizona Press, 1971).

10. Geza Roheim, *Women and Their Life in Central Australia* (London: The Institute, 1933).

11. Maureen Trudelle Schwartz. 1997. *Molded in the Image of Changing Woman: Navajo Views on the Human Body and Personhood.* Tucson: University of Arizona Press.

12. Eileen Jensen Krige, *Girls' Puberty Songs and Their Relation to Fertility, Health, Morality, and Religion Among the Zulus* (London: Oxford University Press, 1968).

13. Jiro Tanaka, *The San, Hunter-Gatherers of the Kalahari: A Study in Ecological Anthropology* (Tokyo: Tokyo University Press, 1980).

7. Some attributes of the breast

1. Elaine Morgan, *The Descent of Woman* (New York: Stein and Day, 1972).

2. Melvin Konner, *Aspects of the Developmental Ecology of a Foraging People* (Cambridge: At the University Press, 1972).

3. Raymond DeCoccola, *The Incredible Eskimo: Life Among the Barren Land Eskimo* (Surrey, BC and Blaine, WA: Hancock House, 1986).

4. Mischa Titiev, *The Hopi Indians of Old Oraibi: Change and Continuity* (Ann Arbor: University of Michigan Press, 1972).

5. Herbert Basedow, *The Australian Aboriginal* (Adelaide: F.W. Preece and Sons, 1925).

6. Ronald Singer, *The Biology of the San* (Cape Town and Pretoria: Human & Rousseau, 1978).

7. Geoffrey Miller, *The Mating Mind: How Sexual Choice Shaped the Evolution of Human Nature*, (New York: Anchor Books, 2001).

8. Beliefs about maturation of the breasts

1. Geoffrey Gorer, and J. H. Hutton, *Himalayan Village: An Account of the Lepchas of Sikkim* (London: Michael Joseph, Ltd, 1938).
2. Thomas Gladwin, and Seymour B. Sarason, *Truk: Man in Paradise* (New York: Wenner Gren Foundation for Anthropological Research, 1953), 110.
3. Ward Hunt Goodenough, *Property, Kin, and Community On Truk* (New Haven: Published for Dept. of Anthropology, Yale University, Yale University Press, 1961).
4. Marc J. Swartz, *Sexuality and Aggression On Romonum, Truk* (Washington: American Anthropological Society, 1958).
5. Zarko David Levak, *Kinship System and Social Structure of the Bororo of Pobojari* (Ann Arbor, Michican: University Microfilms, 1973).
6. Paul Hocking, *Sex and Disease in a Mountain Community* (Sahibabad, Dist. Ghaziabad: Vikas Publishing Pvt. Ltd, 1980).
7. Geza Roheim, *Women and Their Life in Central Australia* (London: The Institute, 1933).

9. The start of a girl's sexual life

1. Ronald Singer, *The Biology of the San* (Cape Town and Pretoria: Human & Rousseau, 1978).
2. A. Stewart Truswell and John D. L. Hansen, *Medical Research Among the !Kung* (Cambridge, Mass: Harvard University Press, 1976).
3. George B. Silberbauer, *The G/wi Bushmen* (New York: Holt, Rinehart and Winston, 1972).
4. Lorna Marshall, *Marriage Among !Kung Bushmen* (London: Oxford University Press, 1959).

5. Marjorie Shostak, *Nisa: The Life and Words of a !KungWoman* (Cambridge, Mass: Harvard University Press, 1981).

6. Peter Sarpong, *Girls' Nobility Rites on Ashanti* (Tema, Ghana: Ghana Pub. Corp, 1977).

7. E. E. Evans-Pritchard, *The Azande: History and Political Institutions* (Oxford: Clarendon Press, 1971).

8. Genevieve Calame-Griaule, *Words and the Dogon World* (Philadelphia: Institute for the Study of Human Issues, 1986).

9. John Roscoe, *The Baganda: An Account of Their Native Customs and Beliefs* (London, Macmillan and Co, 1911).

10. Lucy Philip Mair, *An African People in the Twentieth Century* (London: Routledge & Sons, 1934).

11. Absolom Vilakazi, *Zulu Transformations: A Study of the Dynamics of Social Change* (Pietermaritzburg: University of Natal Press, 1962).

12. Eileen Jensen Krige, *Girls' Puberty Songs and Their Relation to Fertility, Health, Morality, and Religion among the Zulus* (London: Oxford University Press, 1968).

13. Mary Felice Smith, *Baba of Karo, A Woman of the Muslim Hausa* (London: Farber and Farber, 1966).

14. Paul Spencer, *The Maasai of Matapato: A Study of Rituals of Rebellion* (Bloomington, Ind: Indiana University Press, 1988).

15. Charulal Mukherjea, *The Santals* (Calcutta: A. Mukherjee & Co., Private Ltd, 1962). P. 415.

16. Erika Friedl, *Children of Deh Koh: Young Life in an Iranian Village* (Syracuse, NY: Syracuse University Press, 1997).

17. Leopold J. Pospisil, *Kapauku Papuans and Their Law* (New Haven, Conn: Published for the Department of Anthropology, Yale University, 1958).

18. Cora Alice DuBois, Abram Kardiner, and Emil Oberholzer, *The People of Alor: A Social-Psychological Study of An East Indian Island* (Minneapolis: Univ. of Minnesota Press, 1944).

19. Melville Jean Herskovits, *Rebel Destiny: Among the Bush Negroes of Dutch Guiana* (New York: Whittlesey House, McGraw-Hill Book Company, Incorporated, 1934).

10. The breasts and clothing

1. William Kester Barnett, *An Ethnographic Description of Sanlei Ts'un, Taiwan, With Emphasis On Women's Roles: Overcoming Research Problems Caused by the Presence of a Great Tradition* (Ann Arbor Mich: University Microfilms, 1971).
2. Nicolaus Adriani, *The Bare'e-Speakig Torakja of Central Celebes (The East Toradja): Third Volume* (Amsterdam: Noord-Hollandsche Uitgevers Maatschappij, 1951).
3. Helen Morton Lee, *Becoming Tongan: An Ethnography of Childhood* (Honolulu: University of Hawai'i Press, 1996).
4. Gerd Koch, *The South Seas –Yesterday and Today* (New Haven: Human Relations Area Files, 1979).
5. Christine Ward Gailey, "Putting Down Sisters and Wives: Tongan Women and Colonization," in *Women and Colonization,* ed. Mona Etienne and Eleanor Leacock (New York: Praeger, 1980).
6. Audrey Isabel Richards, *Chisungu: A Girls' Initiation Ceremony Among the Bemba of Northern Rhodesia* (London, England: Faber and Faber, 1956).
7. Sally Price, *Co-wives and Calabashes* (Ann Arbor: University of Michigan Press, 1993).
8. Laura W. R. Appell, *Menstruation Among the Rungus: An Unmarked Category,* (Berkeley: University of California Press, 1988).
9. Gerardo Reichel-Dolmatoff, *Amazonian Cosmos: The Sexual and Religious Symbolism of the Tukano Indians* (Chicago: the University of Chicago Press, 1971).

Chapter IV: The breast depicted in myth and the arts

1. Three creation myths

1. Taye Assefa, *Dreams in Amharic Prose Fiction* (Addis Ababa: Haile Selassie University, Institute of Ethiopian Studies, 1988), 173.
2. *Holy Bible: New Catholic Edition* (New York: Catholic Book Publishing Co, 1957).
3. Penny Petrone, ed., *Northern Voices: Inuit Writing in English* (Toronto: University of Toronto Press, 1988).

2. Stories from around the globe

1. Dorothy Demetracopulou Lee, *Greece* (Paris: UNESCO, 1953), 83.
2. Enrico Cerulli, *How a Hawiye Tribe Used To Live* (A Cure dell'Amministrazione Fiduciaria Italiana della Somalia; Instituto poligrafico dello Stato P. V., 1959), 108.
3. Roy Franklin Barton, *The Mythology of the Ifugaos* (Philadelphia: American Folklore Society, 1955), 103.
4. Robert Redfield, *A Village That Chose Progress: Chan Kom Revisited* (Chicago; London: Phoenix Books, The University of Chicago Press, 1962), 116.
5. Alfonso Villa Rojas, *The Maya of East Central Quintana Roo* (Washington, D. C.: Carnegie Institution of Washington, 1945), 152.
6. Allan F. Burns, A*n Epoch of Miracles: Oral Literature of the Yucatec Maya* (Austin: University of Texas Press, 1983), 1983.
7. Robert Redfield, *A Village That Chose Progress: Chan Kom Revisited* (Chicago; London: Phoenix Books, The University of Chicago Press, 1962).
8. Gerardo Reichel-Dolmatoff, *Amazonian Cosmos: The Sexual and Religious Symbolism of the Tukano Indians* (Chicago: the University of Chicago Press, 1971).

9. Egon Schaden and Lars-Peter Lewinsohn, *Fundamental Aspects of Guarani Culture* (Sao Paulo: Difusao Europeia do Livro, 1962), 146.

10. Mischa Titiev, *The Hopi Indians of Old Oraibi: Change and Continuity* (Ann Arbor: University of Michigan Press, 1972).

11. Alexander M. Stephen and Elsie W. C. Parsons, *Hopi Journal of Alexander M. Stephen* (New York. AMS Press, 1969).

12. Geza Roheim, *The Eternal Ones of the Dream: a Psychoanalytic Interpretation of Australian Myth and Ritual* (New York: International Universities Press, 1945), 183.

13. Edwin H.Gomes, *Seventeen Years Among the Sea Dyaks of Borneo: A Record of Intimate Association With the Natives of the Bornean Jungles* (London, England: Seeley & Co. Ltd, 1911), 206.

14. Willard Williams Hill, *The Agricultural and Hunting Methods of the Navaho Indians* (New Haven, London: Published for the Department of Anthropology, Yale University, by the Yale University Press; H. Milford, Oxford University Press, 1938), 99.

15. Grenville Goodwin, *Myths and Tales of the White Mountain Apache* (New York: The American Folk-lore Socity, J. J. Augustin, Agent, 1939).

16. Zarko David Levak, *Kinship System and Social Structure of the Bororo of Pobojari* (Ann Arbor, Michican: University Microfilms, 1973).

17. William George Archer, *The Hill of Flutes: Life, Love, and Poetry in Tribal India: A Portrait of the Santals* (Pittsburgh: University of Pittsburgh Press, 1974).

18. Alfred Metraux and Priscilla Reynolds, *Contributions to Andean folklore* (New Haven, Conn: Human Relations Area Files, 1934), 11.

19. Hilma Natalia Granqvist, *Marriage Conditions in a Palestinian Village: volume 2* (Helsingfors, Finland: Akademische Buchandlung, 1935).

20. Jeremija M. Pavlovic, *Folklife and Customs in the Kragujevac Region of the Jasenica in Sumdaija* (New Haven, Conn: Human Relations Area Files, 1973), 138.

21. Milenko S. Filipovic, *Among the People, Native Yugoslav Ethnography: Selected writings of Milenko S. Filipovic* (Ann Arbor, Mich.: Michigan Slavic Publications, Dept. of Slavic Languages and Literatures, 1982).

22. Henri Masse, *Persian Beliefs and Customs* (New Haven, Conn: Human Relations Area Files, 1954).

23. E.E.Evans-Pritchard, *Witchcraft, Oracles and Magic Among the Azande* (Oxford: Clarendon Press, 1937).

24. Ruy Galvao de Andrade Coelho, *The Black Carib of Honduras: A Study in Acculturation* (Ann Arbor, Mich.: University Microfilms, 1955), 149.

25. Robert A. Paul, *The Tibetan Symbolic World: Psychoanalytic Explorations* (Chicago: University of Chicago Press, 1982), 148.

Chapter V: Women's sexuality: some history and pre-history

1. The breasts and religion

1. Joseph Campbell, *The Masks of God: Primitive Mythology* (New York: Arkana, Penguin Books, 1991).

2. Nicholas J. Conard, "A Female Figurine From the Basal Aurignacian of Hohle Fels Cave in Southwestern Germany," *Nature* 459 (7244) (May 14, 2009): 248-252.

3. Marija Gimbutas, *The Language of the Goddess* (San Francisco: Harper & Row, 1989), figure 53, p.35: bird-woman hybrid with arm supporting her breast; 5900 – 5700 BC. Sesklo (Megali Vrisi, Timavos), Thessaly.

4. Anne Baring and Jules Cashford, *The Myth of the Goddess: Evolution of an Image* (New York: Viking Arkana, Penguin Books, 1991).

5. Marion McCreedy, "The Arms of the Dibouka," in *Key Issues In Hunter-Gatherer Research*, ed. Ernest S. Burch, Jr. and Linda J. Ellanna (Oxford UK: Berg Press, 1994).

6. Anne Baring and Jules Cashford, *The Myth of the Goddess: Evolution of an Image* (New York: Viking Arkana, Penguin Books, 1991), figure 16, p. 198: Ishtar as goddess of fertility; c. 2000 BC.

7. Marilyn Yalom, *A History of the Breast*. (New York: Alfred A. Knopf, 1997), 11.

8. Anne Baring and Jules Cashford, *The Myth of the Goddess, Evolution of an Image* (New York: Viking Arkana, Penguin Books, 1991), figure 8, p. 455: image of the goddess Asherah or Astarte, unglazed earthenware; seventh century BC. Tell Duweir, Palestine.

9. Anne Baring and Jules Cashford, in *The Myth of the Goddess, Evolution of an Image* (New York: Viking Arkana, Penguin Books, 1991), figure 5, p. 314: the sacred marriage of Hera and Zeus, wood carving; late seventh century BCE; possibly from Samos.

10. Anne Baring and Jules Cashford, in *The Myth of the Goddess, Evolution of an Image* (New York: Viking Arkana, Penguin Books, 1991), figure 29, p. 214: marriage bed with embracing couple, clay plaque; c. 2000 BC. Elam, present day Southwest Iran.

11. Anne Baring and Jules Cashford, *The Myth of the Goddess, Evolution of an Image* (New York: Viking Arkana, Penguin Books, 1991), figure 22, p. 67: sculpted figure showing the Goddess giving birth to a snake and suckling it; date unknown, possible Gallo-Roman. The village of Oo in the Luchon region of the Pyrenees, south-Western France.

12. Marilyn Yalom, *A History of the Breast* (New York: Alfred A. Knopf, 1997), figure 6, p. 14: gold-and-ivory snake goddess; c.1500 – 1600 BCE, Minoan (Crete).

13. Marilyn Yalom, *A History of the Breast* (New York: Alfred A. Knopf, 1997), figure 13, p. 33: church fresco; early twelfth century, Tavant, France.

14. Francis Haskell and Nicholas Penny, *Taste and the Antique: the Lure of Classical Sculpture, 1500-1900.* (New Haven: Yale University Press, 1981), figure 173, p.327: Venus de' Medici; probably from the first century BC.

15. Elaine G. Breslaw, ed., *Witches of the Atlantic World: A Historical Reader and Primary Sourcebook* (New York: New York University Press, 2000), introduction.

16. Anne Llewellyn Barstow, *Witchcraze* (San Francisco: Pandora/Harper Collins, 1994), 21.

17. Matthew Hopkins, "The Discovery of Witches," in *Witches of the Atlantic World: A Historical Reader and Primary Sourcebook,* ed. Elaine G. Breslaw (New York: New York University Press, 2000).

18. Anne Llewellyn Barstow, *Witchcraze* (San Francisco: Pandora/Harper Collins, 1994), 144.

19. Heinrich Kramer and Jacob Sprenger, "Why Women Are Chiefly Addicted to Evil Superstitions," in *Witches of the Atlantic World: A Historical Reader & Primary Sourcebook,* ed. Elaine G. Breslaw (New York: New York University Press, 2000).

2. The uterus and medicine

1. Helen King, *Hippocrates' Woman: Reading the Female Body in Ancient Greece* (New York: Routledge, 1989).

2. Helen King, "OnceUupon a Text: Hysteria From Hippocrates," in *Hysteria Beyond Freud* by Sander L. Gilman, Helen King, G.S. Rousseau, Roy Porter, and Elaine Showalter (Berkeley: University of California Press, 1993).

3. William H. Masters and Virginia Johnson, *The Human Sexual Response.* (London: J. & A. Churchhill, Ltd, 1966).

4. Regina Morantz-Sanchez, *Conduct Unbecoming a Woman: Medicine on Trial in Turn-of-the- Century Brooklyn* (New York: Oxford University Press, 1999).
5. William H. Parker M.D. and Rachel L. Parker, *A Gynecologist's Second Opinion: The Questions and Answers You Need To Take Charge of Your Life* (New York: Penguin, 1996).
6. J.M. Wu, M.E. Wechter, E.J. Geller, T.V. Nguyen, and A.G. Visco. "Hysterectomy Rates in the United States, 2003," *Obstet Gynecol* 110 (5) (2007): 1091-1095.
7. Marcia G. Kramer, P.A. and Robert C. Reiter, M.D., "Hysterectomy: Indications, Alternatives and Predictors," *American Family Physician* 55(3) (Feb, 1997): 827-834.
8. HERS Foundation, 422 Bryn Mawr Avenue, Bala Cynwyd, PA 19004.
9. Bruce M. Carlson, MD, PhD, *Patten's Foundations of Embryology, Fifth Edition* (New York: McGraw-Hill, 1988), 575.

Chapter VI: Sexual pleasure, sociality, and happiness

1. Orgasm and equality between the sexes

1. Desmond Morris, *The Naked Ape: A Zoologist's Study of the Human Animal* (New York, McGraw-Hill, 1967).
2. Jane Goodall, *The Chimpanzees of Gombe* (Cambridge, Massachusetts: The Belknap Press of Harvard University Press, 1986).
3. D.A. Goldfoot, H. Westerborg-vanLoon, W. Groenveld, and A.K. Slob. "Behavioral and Physiological Evidence of Sexual Climax in the Female StumpTtailed Macaque (*Macaca arctoides*)," *Science* 208 (4451) (Jun 27, 1980): 1477-9.
4. F.D. Burton, "Sexual Climax in Female *Macaca mulatta*," in *Proceedings of the Third International Congress of Primatology* (Basel: Karger, 1971).

5. S. Chevalier-Skolnikoff, "Male-Female, Female-Female, and Male-Male Sexual Behavior in the Stumptail Monkey With Special Attention to the Female Orgasm," *Archives of Sexual Behavior:* 3 (1974): 95-116.

6. Frans B.M. deWaal, *Peacekeeping Among Primates* (Cambridge: Harvard University Press, 1989).

7. Mary S. McDonald Pavelka, "Sexual Nature: What Can We Learn From a Cross-Species Perspective?" in *Sexual Nature: Sexual Culture,* ed. Paul R. Abramson and Steven D. Pinkerton (Chicago and London: The University of Chicago Press, 1995).

8. Leonard Shlain, *Sex, Ttime, and Power: How Women's Sexuality Shaped Human Evolution* (New York: Viking Adult, Penguin, 2003).

9. Donald Symons, *The Evolution of Human Sexuality* (New York: Oxford University Press, 1979), 82.

10. Shere Hite, *The Hite Report: A Nationwide Study of Female Sexuality* (New York: Seven Stories Press, 2004).

11. Frans B. M. deWaal, "Sex As an Alternative to Aggression in the Bonobo," in *Sexual Nature: Sexual Culture,* ed. Paul R. Abramson and Steven D. Pinkerton (Chicago and London: The University of Chicago Press, 1995).

12. Paul R. Abramson and Steven D. Pinkerton, *With Pleasure: Thoughts On the Nature of Human Sexuality* (New York: Oxford University Press, 2000).

13. Frans B. M. deWaal, Cited above.

14. Philip Lieberman, *Eve spoke: Human Language and Human Evolution* (New York: W. W. Norton, 1998).

15. Christopher Boehm, *Hierarchy in the Forest* (Cambridge, MA: Harvard University Press, 1999), 173.

16. Eleanor Burke Leacock, *Myths of Male Dominance: Collected Articles on Women Cross-Culturally* (New York and London: Monthly Review Press, 1981), 35.

2. Cultural sexuality: positive emotions and sociality

1. Donald Symons, *The Evolution of Human Sexuality* (New York: Oxford University Press, 1979).
2. J. Bancroft, "The Endocrinology of Sexual Arousal," *The Journal of Endocrinology* 186(3) (September, 2005): 411-27.
3. Nicholas Christakis and James H. Fowler, "Dynamic Spread of Happiness in a Large Social Network: Longitudinal Analysis Over 20 years in the Framingham Heart Study," *British Medical Journal 337 no. a2338* (December, 2008): 1-9.
4. John T. Cacioppo, "Strangers May Cheer You Up, Study Says". *New York Times International,* Friday, December 5, 2008. www.nytimes-com/2008/12/05/health/05happy-web. html
5. Robin Allott, "Evolutionary Aspects of Love and Empathy," *Journal of Social and Evolutionary Systems* 15, no. 4 (1992): 353-370.
6. Herbert Spencer, *Social Statics. The Conditions Essential to Human Happiness Specified, and One of Them Developed* (New York: D. Appleton and Co, 1890), 226.
7. Thomas Gregor, "Sexuality and the Experience of Love," in *Sexual Nature Sexual Culture,* ed. Paul R Abramson and Steven D. Pinkerton (Chicago: The University of Chicago Press, 1995), 333.
8. W. K. Jankowiak and E. F. Fischer, "A Cross-Cultural Perspective on Romantic Love," *Ethnology* 31(2) (1992): 149.

3. Happiness and human development

1. Theodore D. Kemper, "How Many Emotions Are There? Wedding the Social and Autonomic Components," *American Journal of Sociology* 93, no. 2 (Sept, 1987): 263-289.
2. Jonathan H. Turner, *On the Origin of Human Emotions: A Sociological Inquiry Into the Evolution of Human Affect* (Stanford, CA: Stanford University Press, 2000).
3. Zoltan Kovecses, *Emotion Concepts* (New York: Springer-Verlag, 1990), 141.

4. Barbara L. Fredrickson, "What Good Are Positive Emotions" *Review of General Psychology* 2, no. 3 (1998): 300-319.

5. Annette Bolte, Thomas Goschke, and Julius Kuhl, "Emotion and Intuition: Effects of Positive and Negative Mood in Implicit Judgments of Semantic Coherence," *Psychological Science* 14, no. 5. (September, 2003): 416-421.

6. Herbert Spencer, *Social Statics. The Conditions Essential to Human Happiness Specified, and One of Them Developed* (London: John Chapman, 1851), 203.

7. Robert J. Sternberg, "A Triangular Theory of Love." *Psychological Review* 93, no.2 (2007): 119-135.

8. Thomas Gregor, "Sexuality and the Experience of Love," in *Sexual Nature Sexual Culture,* ed. Paul R. Abramson and Steven D. Pinkerton (Chicago: The University of Chicago Press, 1995), 333.

9. William F. Hanks, "Joint Commitment and Common Ground in a Ritual Event," in *Roots of Human Sociality: Culture, Cognition, and Interaction,* ed. N.J. Enfield and Stephen C. Levinson (New York: Berg, 2006).

10. Herbert H. Clark and Susan E. Brennan, "Grounding in Communication," in *Perspectives on Socially Shared Cognition,* ed. Lauren B. Resnick, John M. Levine, and Stephanie D. Teasley (Washington D.C.: American Psychological Association, 1991).

4. Past and present

1. A. C. Kinsey and the Staff of the Institute for Sex Research, Indiana University, *Sexual Behavior of the Human Female* (Philadelphia: W. B.Saunders, 1953).

2. Shere Hite, *The Hite Report: a Nationwide Study of Female Sexuality* (New York: Seven Stories Press, 2004).

3. L.S.Vygotsky, *Mind In Society: The Development of Higher Psychological Processes* (Cambridge MA: Harvard University Press, 1978).

4. Johan Lind and Patrik Lindenfore, "The Number of Cultural Traits is Correlated with Female Group Size but Not with Male Group Size in Chimpanzee Communities," *PLoS ONE 5(3): e9241* (March 2010) DOI☐: 10.1371/journal. pone.0009241.
5. Donald S. Marshall, "Sexual Behavior on Mangaia," in *Human Sexual Behavior,* ed. D.S. Marshall and R.C. Suggs (New York: Basic Books, 1971).
6. Antonio R. Damasio, *Descartes' Error: Emotion, Reason, and the Human Brain.* New York: Putnam, 1994), 176-177.
7. William H. Calvin, *A Brief History of the Mind: From Ape to Intellect and Beyond* (New York: Oxford University Press, 2004).

Chapter VII: Women's health

1. Sexual dysfunction, depression, and cancer

1. E. O. Laumann, A. Paik, R. C. Rosen, "Sexual Dysfunction in the United States: Prevalence and Predictors," *JAMA* 281(6) (Feb 10, 1999): 537-544.
2. E. McGrath, G. P. Keita, B. R. Strickland, and N. Russo, *Women and Depression: Risk Factors and Treatment Issues* (Washington DC: American Psychological Association, 1990).
3. American Psychological Association, *Research Agenda in Psychosocial and Behavioral Factors in Women's Health. Feb. 1996.* Website: http://www.apa.org/about/gr/issues/women/ depression.aspx Accessed June 15, 2015.
4. D. Herbenick, M. Reese, V. Schick, S. A. Sanders, B. Dodge, J. D. Fortenberry. "Sexual Behavior in the United States: Results From a National Probability Sample of Men and Women Ages 14-94. *J Sex Med* 7 (suppl 5) (2010): 255-265.
5. Gynecologic Cancers Portfolio Analyses Nov. 2012. National Cancer Institute, National Institute of Health, U. S. Department of Health and Human Services. Website: http://

www.icrpartnership.org/Publications/ICRP_GYN_analysis. pdf Accessed June 15, 2015.

6. K. E. Brock, G. Berry, and L. A. Brinton, "Sexual, Reproductive and Contraceptive Risk Factors For Carcinoma-in-situ of the Uterine Cervix in Sydney," *Med J of Aust* 50 (1989): 125-130.

7. P. A. Newcomb and A. Trentham-Dietz. "Breast Feeding Practices in Relation to Endometrial Cancer Risk, USA," *Cancer Causes Control* 11 (Aug, 2000): 663-7.

8. David A. Grimes and K. E. Economy, "Primary Prevention of Gynecologic Cancers," *Am J Obstet Gynecol* 172 (1995): 227-235.

9. Susan G. Komen. Website: http://ww5.komen.org/ BreastCancer/Statistics.html Accessed June 15, 2015.

10. N. Howlader, A. M. Noone, M. Krapcho, et al, eds., *SEER Cancer Statistics Review, 1975-2012.* (Bethesda, MD: National Cancer Institute, 2012). http://www.seer.cancer. gov/statfacts/html/breast.html Go to Trends in Rates. Accessed June 15, 2015.

11. Valerie Beral and the Collaborative Group on Hormonal Factors in Breast Cancer. "Breast Cancer and Breast Feeding Collaborative Reanalysis of Individual Data From 47 Epidemiological Studies in 30 Countries, Including 50,302 Women With Breast Cancer and 96,973 Women Without the Disease," *Lancet* 360 (2002):187-195.

12. Timothy G. C. Murrell. Epidemiological and biochemical support for a theory on the cause and prevention of breast cancer. *Medical Hypotheses* 36 (1991): 389-396.

2. To find a cure, look within

1. N. Howlader, A.M. Noone, M. Krapcho, et al (eds), *SEER Cancer Statistics Review, 1975-2009, Vintage 2009 Populations* (Bethesda, MD: National Cancer Institute, 2012)

2. J. S. Mandelblatt, K. A. Cronin, S. Bailey, et al., "Effects of Mammography Screening Under Different Screening

Schedules: Model Estimates of Potential Benefits and Harms," *Annals of Internal Medicine* 151(10) (2009): 738-747.
3. A.B. Mariotto, K.R. Yabroff, Y. Shao, E.J. Feuer, and M.L. Brown,. "Projections of the Cost of Cancer Care in the United States: 2010 – 2020," *Journal of the National Cancer Institute* 103, no. 2 (2011): 117-128. doi: 10.1093/jnci/djq49
4. American Cancer Society. 2011- 2012. *Cancer Facts and Figures 2011-2012.* Atlanta: American Cancer Society.
5. American Cancer Society. *Cancer Facts and Figures 2012.* (Atlanta: American Cancer Society, 2012).
6. "From Cause to Cure, A Special Advertising Supplement to the New York Times Magazine." *The New York Times Magazine,* October 10, 1999.

3. Breastfeeding

1. *National Immunization Survey.* (Atlanta, GA: Center for Disease Control and Prevention (CDC), 2013).
2. *Ross Laboratories Mothers' Survey* (Columbus, OH: Ross Laboratories, 2000).
3. Elizabeth N. Baldwin, "Extended Breastfeeding and the Law," *Breastfeeding Abstracts* 20, no. 3 (Feb, 2001):19-20.
4. American Academy of Pediatrics, "Breastfeeding and the Use of Human milk." *Pediatrics* 100 (Dec, 1997): 1035-1039.
5. Mary D. (Salter) Ainsworth, *Infancy in Uganda: Infant Care and the Growth of Love* (Baltimore: John Hopkins Press, 1967).
6. Robert Alan LeVine, Sarah Levine, P. Herbert Leiderman, T. Berry Brazelton, Suzanne Dixon, Amy Richman, Constance H. Keefer, James Caron, Rebecca Staples New, Patrice Miller, Edward Tronick, David Feigal, and Jos Yaman. *Variations in Infant Interaction: Illustrative Cases* (Cambridge; Cambridge University Press, 1994).

4. Women build a movement

1. American Academy of Pediatrics. 1997. "Breastfeeding and the Use of Human Milk," *Pediatrics* 100 (Dec, 1997): 1035-1039.
2. La Leche League International and Diane Wiessinger, Diana West, Teresa Pitman. *The Womanly Art of Breastfeeding: Completely Revised and Updated 8th Edition* (New York: Ballantine Books, 2010).
3. The Boston Women's Health Book Collective and author Judy Norsigian. *Our Bodies, Ourselves: A New Edition for a New Era* (New York: Touchstone Books, 2005).
4. Jacque Wilson. From 'filthy trash' to 'iconic resource': *Our Bodies, Ourselves* at 40. http://www.cnn.com/2011/10/05/health/our-bodies-ourselves-40thanniversary/index.html Accessed August 2016.
5. Gale Pryor *Nursing Mother, Working Mother* (Boston: The Harvard Common Press, 1997).

5. Prevention

1. Valerie Beral and the Collaborative Group on Hormonal Factors in Breast Cancer, "Breast Cancer and Breast Feeding Collaborative Reanalysis of Individual Data From 47 Epidemiological Studies in 30 Countries, Including 50,302 Women With Beast Cancer and 96,973 Women Without the Disease," *The Lancet* 360 (2002): Beral187-195.
2. K.G. Auerbach, and J.L. Avery, "Induced Lactation: A Study of Adoptive Nursing by 240 Women." *American journal of diseases in children* 135 (4) (Apr, 1981): 340-3.
3. Isabelle Romieu, "Breast Cancer and Lactation History in Mexican Women," *American Journal of Epidemiology* 143 (1966): 543-552.
4. Tongzhang Zheng, L. Duan, Y. Liu, B. Zhang, Y. Wang, Y. Chen, Y. Zhang, P.H. Owens, "Lactation Reduces Breast Cancer Risk in Shandong Province, China," *American Journal of Epidemiology,* 152 (2000): 1129-1135.

5. Keun-Young Yoo, K. Tagima, T. Kuroishi, K. Hirose, M. Yoshida, S. Miura, H. Murai, "Independent Protective Effect of Lactation Against Breast Cancer: A Case-Control Study in Japan," *American Journal of Epidemiology* 135 (1992): 726-733.

6. Roy Ing, N.L. Petrakis, J.H. Ho, "Unilateral Breast-Feeding and Breast Cancer," *The Lancet* 2 (July, 1977): 124-127.

7. C. Biancifiori, G.M. Bonser, F. Caschera "Chemically Induced Mammary Tumours Following Unilateral Excision of the Nipples in Pseudo-Pregnant and Lactating Breeding BALB/c Mice," *British Journal of Cancer* 16 (1962): 232-7.

8. H. Furberg, B. Newman, P. Moorman, R. Millikan "Lactation and Breast Cancer Risk," *International Journal of Epidemiology* 28 (1999): 396-402.

9. Cornelius Knabbe, M.E. Lippman, L.M. Wakefield, K.C. Flanders, A. Kasid, R. Derynck, R. B. Dickson, "Evidence That Transforming Growth Factor-B Is a Hormonally Regulated Negative Growth Factor in Human Breast Cancer Cells," *Cell* 48 (1987): 417-428.

10. E. Dewailly, P. Ayotte, J. Brisson, "Protective Effect of Breast Feeding on Breast Cancer and Body Burden of Carcinogenic Organochlorines," *Journal of the National Cancer Institute* 86 (May, 1994): 803 Correspondence.

11. Polly A. Newcomb, et al., "Lactation In Relation To Postmenopausal Breast Cancer," *American Journal of Epidemiology* 150 (1999): 174-182.

12. American Academy of Pediatrics, "Breastfeeding and the Use of Human Milk," *Pediatrics* 100 (Dec, 1997): 1035-1039.

6. Science, education, and the sexual breast

1. Walter B. Quisenberry, "Sociocultural Factors in Cancer in Hawaii," *Annals of the New York Academy of Sciences* 84 (1960): 795-806.

2. The Kinsey Institute: Frequently asked Questions to the Kinsey Institute www.indiana.edu/~kinsey/resources/FAQ.html Accessed August 2015.

3. L. Hanson, J. Mann, S. McMahon, and T. Wong, "Sexual Health," *BMC Women's Health*, 4 (suppl1) (2004): s24.

4. D. Herbenick, M. Reese, V. Schick, S. A. Sanders, B. Dodge, and J. D. Fortenberry. "Sexual Behavior in the United States: Results From a National Probability Sample of Men and Women Ages 14-94," *J Sex Med 7 (suppl 5) (2010): 255-265*.

5. R. Levin and C. Meston. "Nipple/Breast Stimulation and Sexual Arousal in Young Men and Women," *J Sex Med* 3(3) (2006): 450-454.

6. Susanna Schrobsdorff. "Anxiety, Depression, and the American Adolescent," *Time:* November 7, 2016.

7. D. J. Landry, S. Singh, J. E. Darroch. "Sexuality Education in Fifth and Sixth Grades in U.S. Public Schools," *Family Planning Perspectives* 32(5) (2000): 212-219.

8. Timothy G. C. Murrell, "The Potential for Oxytocin (OT) To Prevent Breast Cancer: A Hypothesis," *Breast Cancer Research and Treatment* 35 (1995): 225-229.

9. J. M. Anderson and D. Etches, "Prevention and Management of Postpartum Hemorrhage," *American Family Physician* 75(6) (Mar 15, 2007): 875-882.

10. S. Chua, S. Arulkumaran, I. Lim, N. Selamat, S.S. Ratnam, "Influence of Breastfeeding and Nipple Stimulation on Postpartum Uterine Activity." *British Journal of Obstetrics and Gynecology* 101 (Sept, 1994): 804-805.

11. Helen King, *Hippocrates' Woman: Reading the Female Body in Ancient Greece* (New York: Routledge, 1989).

12. Jay M. Cooper and Marvin L. Erickson, "Global Endometrial Ablation Technologies," *Obstetrics and Gynecology Clinics of North America* 27, no. 2 (June, 2000): 385.

13. Kaye E. Brock, G. Berry, and L. A. Brinton, "Sexual, Reproductive and Contraceptive Risk Factors For

Carcinoma-In-Situ of the Uterine Cervix in Sydney," *The Medical Journal of Australia* 50 (1989): 125-130.

14. P.A. Newcomb and A. Trentham-Dietz, "Breast Feeding Practices In Relation To Endometrial Cancer Risk, USA," *Cancer Causes Control* 11 (Aug, 2000): 663-7.

15. David A. Grimes and Katherine E. Economy, "Primary Prevention of Gynecologic Cancers," *American Journal of Obstetrics and Gynecology* 172 (1995): 227-235.

List of Illustrations

Printed in the United States
By Bookmasters